Quick Hits in Emergency Medicine

Brandon Allen • Latha Ganti
Bobby Desai

Quick Hits in Emergency Medicine

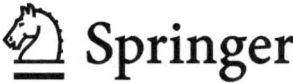 Springer

Brandon Allen, MD
Department of Emergency Medicine
University of Florida
College of Medicine
Gainesville, Florida
USA

Bobby Desai, MD, FACEP
Department of Emergency Medicine
University of Florida
College of Medicine
Gainesville, Florida
USA

Latha Ganti, MD, MS, MBA, FACEP
Departments of Emergency Medicine and Neurological Surgery
Center for Brain Injury Research and Education
University of Florida
College of Medicine
Gainesville, Florida
USA

ISBN 978-1-4614-7036-6   ISBN 978-1-4614-7037-3   (eBook)
DOI 10.1007/978-1-4614-7037-3
Springer New York Heidelberg Dordrecht London

Library of Congress Control Number: 2013943125

Printed on acid-free paper

Springer is part of Springer Science+Business Media (www.springer.com)

To our families—
Nila, Owen, and Katie [Brandon Allen]
Thor, Tej, Trilok, Karthik, Pratik, Mom and
    Dad [Latha Ganti]
Jayden, Dylan, Shayan, and Alpa [Bobby Desai]
                    for the time this endeavor took
                                away from them

To our patients and colleagues—
                    from whom we learn everyday

Contents

1
ACLS

B. Allen et al., *Quick Hits in Emergency Medicine*,
DOI 10.1007/978-1-4614-7037-3_1,
© Springer Science+Business Media New York 2013

ACLS

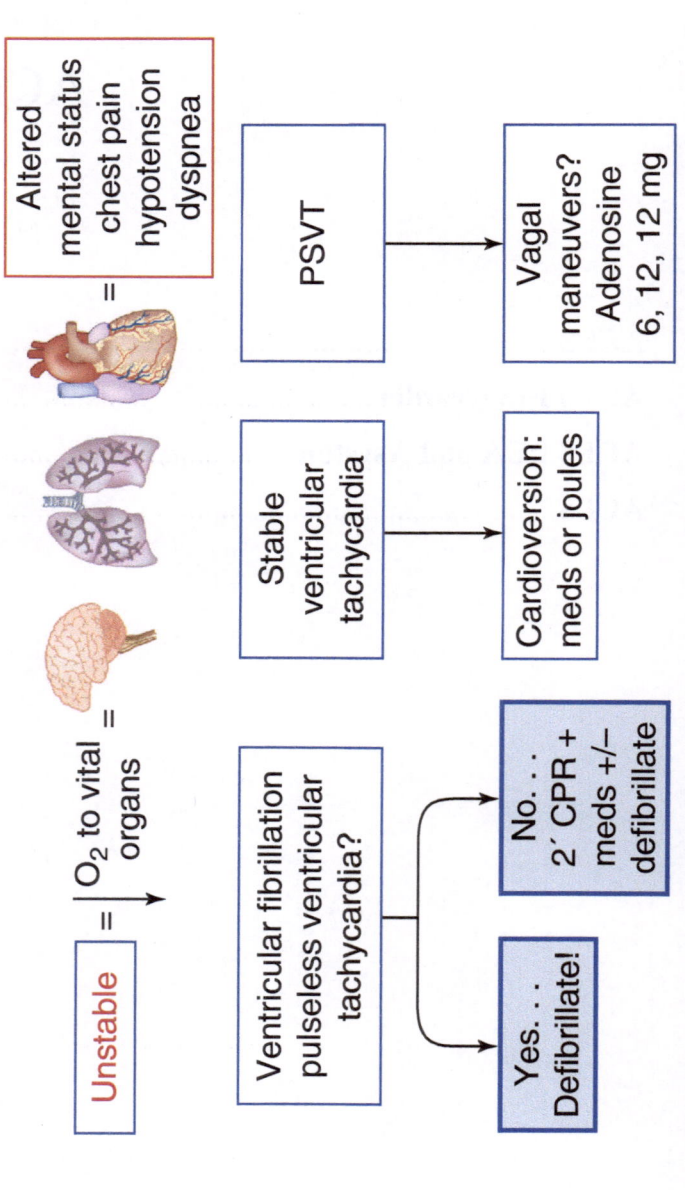

Unstable = | ↓ O_2 to vital organs | =

Altered mental status
chest pain
hypotension
dyspnea

PSVT → Vagal maneuvers? Adenosine 6, 12, 12 mg

Stable ventricular tachycardia → Cardioversion: meds or joules

Ventricular fibrillation pulseless ventricular tachycardia?
→ Yes... Defibrillate!
→ No... 2′ CPR + meds +/– defibrillate

ACLS Bradycardia

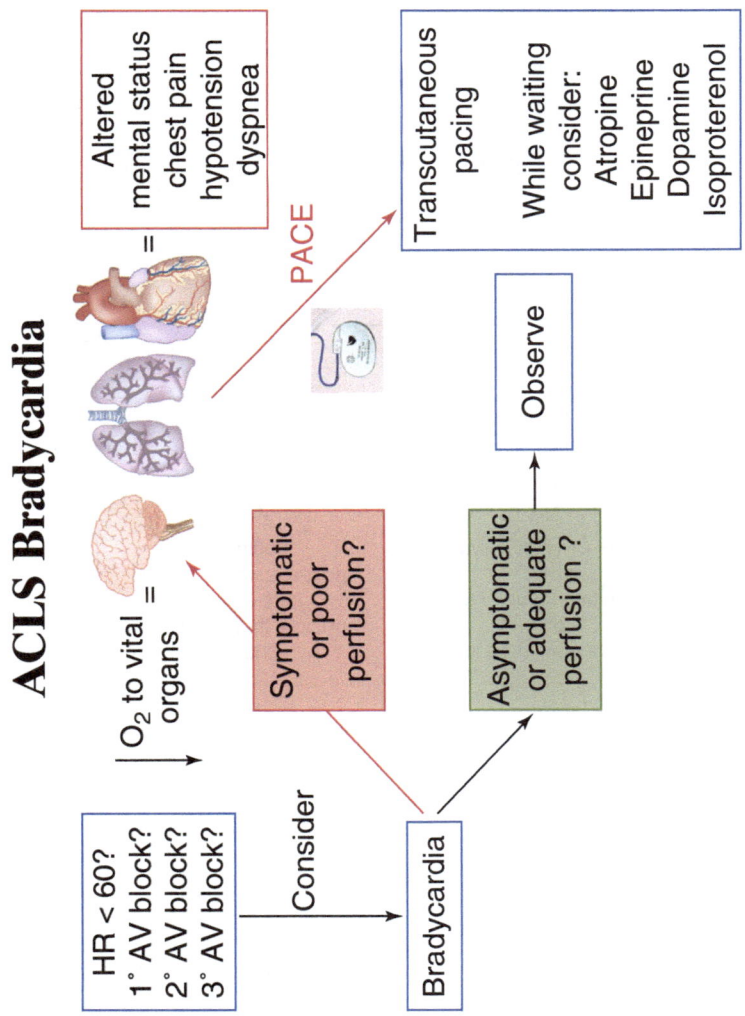

HR < 60?
1° AV block?
2° AV block?
3° AV block?

Consider

O_2 to vital organs =

Bradycardia

Symptomatic or poor perfusion?

Asymptomatic or adequate perfusion ?

Observe

Altered mental status chest pain hypotension dyspnea

PACE

Transcutaneous pacing

While waiting consider:
Atropine
Epineprine
Dopamine
Isoproterenol

ACLS PEA and Asystole

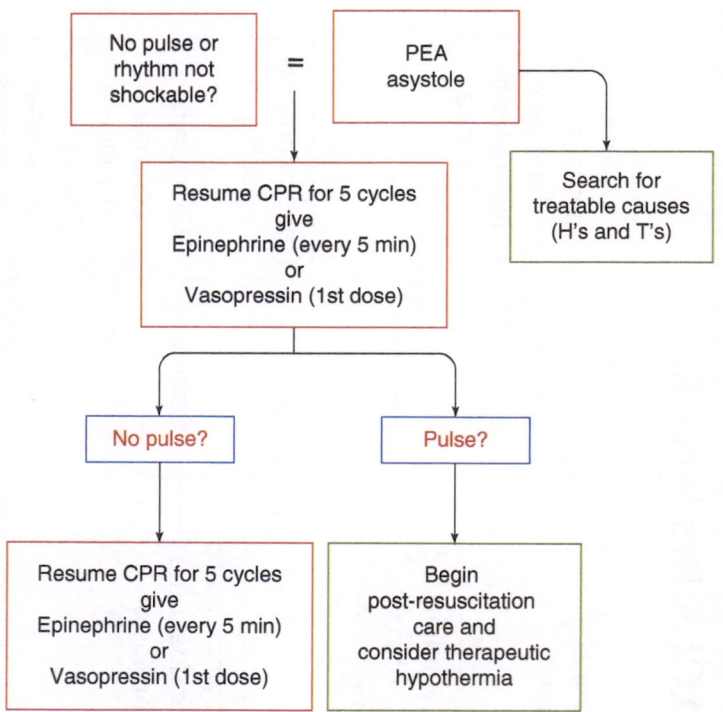

ACLS

- V-Fib

  - Witnessed – shock
  - Unwitnessed – 2 min CPR + meds→shock

- Ventricular tachycardia/paroxysmal supraventricular tachycardia: stable or unstable?

- Electromechanical dissociation/pulseless electrical activity? Think H's and T's

- Heart block/bradycardia: hypotensive?

- Three things that improve survival:

  - Early shock in VF
  - Good compressions
  - Less ventilation

- Adenosine Quick Hits:

  - Never give if HR <150
  - Never give if irregular (A-fib)
  - Never give if vagal maneuvers work to slow HR
  - Beware h/o CHF, COPD, WPW

H's	T's
Hypovolemia	Cardiac tamponade
Hypoxia	Toxins
Hyper or hypokalemia	Thrombosis (cardiac or pulmonary)
Hydrogen ion (acidosis)	Tension pneumothorax
Hypoglycemia	Trauma

2

Intubation, Airway, and Mechanical Ventilation

B. Allen et al., *Quick Hits in Emergency Medicine,*
DOI 10.1007/978-1-4614-7037-3_2,
© Springer Science+Business Media New York 2013

Intubation/Airway

7 P's

- Prepare = equipment
- Pretreat = drugs
- Position = sniffing position (if possible)
- Preoxygenate = 100 % pulse ox (consider apneic oxygenation during direct laryngoscopy) [1]
- Paralyze = drugs
- Placement = tube through cords
- Position = confirm with ETC02 then CXR

1. Weingart, S and Levitan, R. Preoxygenation and prevention of desaturation during emergency airway management. Ann Emerg Med. 2012 Mar; 59(3):165–175

Intubation/Airway

Difficult to Bag

- Obesity
- Beard
- No teeth
- Old/elderly (>55)

Difficult to Intubate (LEMONS)

- **Look externally**
  - Beard? Trauma? Obesity?
- **Evaluate**
  - 3 fingers mouth opening
  - 3 fingers chin to hyoid
  - 2 fingers hyoid to thyroid
- **Mallampati**
  - Classes I–IV
- **Obstruction**
- **Neck mobility**
  - Cervical precautions
- **Saturations**
  - Oxygen reserve

Intubation/Airway

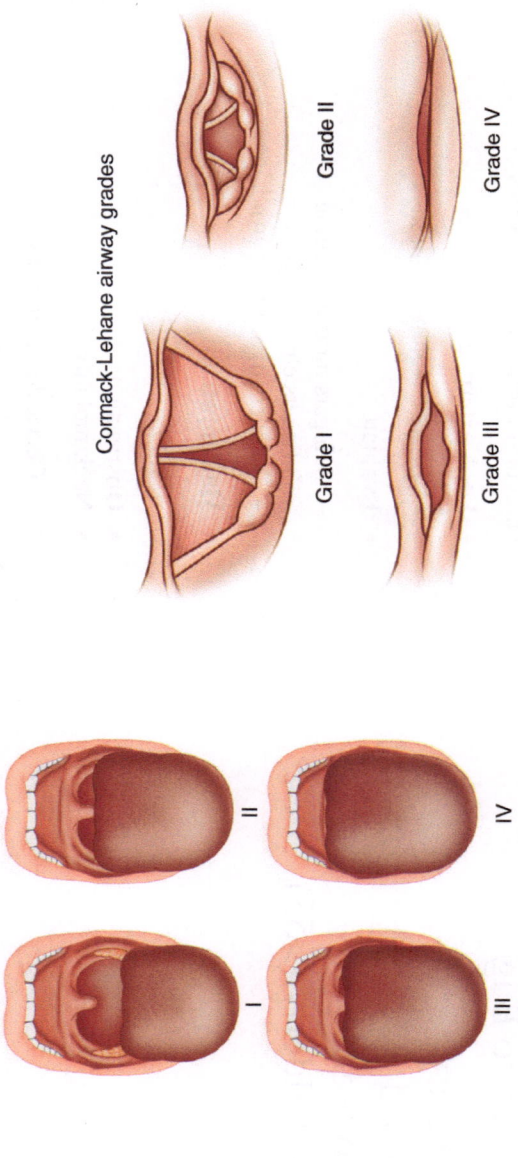

Mallampati score

Cormack-Lehane airway grades

Grade I   Grade II

Grade III   Grade IV

I   II

III   IV

Adapted from: Mallampati SR, Gatt SP, Gugino LD, et al. A clinical sign to predict difficult tracheal intubation: a prospective study. Can Anaesth Soc J 1985;32:429–34

Adapted from: Cormack RS, Lehane J. Difficult tracheal intubation in obstetrics. Cormack-Lehane Airway Grades Anaesthesia 1984; 39: 1105–11

Mechanical Ventilation

	Normal lungs	Asthma/ COPD	ARDS	Hypovolemia
Tidal volume (mL/kg)	8.0	6.0	6.0	8.0
RR	10–12	5–8	10–12	10–12
I/E ratio	1:2	1:4	1:2	1:2
PEEP	4.0	4.0	4–15	0–4
FiO_2	1.0	1.0	1.0	1.0

3

Sepsis and Resuscitation

B. Allen et al., *Quick Hits in Emergency Medicine*,
DOI 10.1007/978-1-4614-7037-3_3,
© Springer Science+Business Media New York 2013

Systemic Inflammatory Response Syndrome (SIRS) and Sepsis

SIRS diagnosis requires two or more to be present

Body temperature <36 or >38

HR >90

RR >20 or $PaCO_2$ <32

WBC <4,000 or >12,000 OR bands >10 %

Sepsis is SIRS with clinical confirmed/suspected infection

Severe sepsis is sepsis and hypotension (that responds to fluids), organ dysfx, hypoperfusion

Septic shock is severe sepsis with refractory hypotension after fluid resuscitation

Early Goal-Directed Therapy

Give Antibiotics Early!

Goal	Therapy
CVP 8–12	Fluid bolus 500 cc Q30 min
	CVP goal 12–15 if mechanically ventilated
MAP >65	Begin prossors/vasoactive agents
$ScvO_2$ >70	Transfuse to Hct >30
	Start inotrope (dobutamine)

Adapted from Rivers E et al. Early goal-directed therapy in the treatment of severe sepsis and septic shock. N Engl J. Med. 2001 Nov 8;345(19):1368–77

Hemodynamics

- Arterial content = (1.34)(Hgb)(arterial sat.)

- Venous content = (1.34)(Hgb)(SVO_2%)

- A-V O_2 Diff. = Art. Content − Venous content

- O_2-Delivery = (Art. Content)(C.O.)(10)

- O_2-Consumption = (A-V O_2 Diff)(C.O.)(10)

- Extraction = A-V O_2 Diff/Arterial Content × 100

4

Pulmonary Decision Rules and COPD

B. Allen et al., *Quick Hits in Emergency Medicine*, 17
DOI 10.1007/978-1-4614-7037-3_4,
© Springer Science+Business Media New York 2013

CURB + CURB-65 Community-Acquired Pneumonia (CAP) Scores

Characteristic	CURB-65 points	CURB points
Confusion	1	1
Urea (BUN >19)	1	1
Respiratory rate >30/min	1	1
Blood pressure (systolic BP<90 or diastolic BP <60)	1	1
Age >65	1	N/A

Adapted from Lim WS, van der Eerden MM, Laing R, et al. (2003) Defining community acquired pneumonia Severity on presentation to hospital: a international derivation and validation study. Thorax 58(5):377–82. N Patients with CURB-65 = 2 or CURB = 1 should be considered for inpatient care or intensive outpatient tx; if hypoxia or hypotension, admit regardless of score

Pulmonary Embolism Rule-Out Criteria (PERC)

PERC (BREATHS) criteria

B – Blood in sputum

R – Room air sat <95 %

E – Estrogen or hormone use

A – Age >50 years

T – Thrombosis in past (DVT, PE) or possible DVT/swollen calf

H – Heart rate >100 beats/min

S – Surgery in past 4 weeks

<u>Inclusion criteria</u>   Suspicion of PE low enough that clinician would be confident enough to exclude if they had normal D-dimer (low-risk group which comprises a population with 8 % PE risk)

Patient(s) with dyspnea BUT PE was not felt to be the most likely diagnosis (very low-risk group—2 % overall PE risk)

<u>Exclusion criteria</u>   DO NOT use this rule if PE suspicion high enough that you would not be confident in excluding PE with a normal D-dimer

Adapted from Kline JA, et al. Prospective multicenter evaluation of the pulmonary embolism rule-out criteria. J Thromb Haemost 2008; 6; 772–80

If all PERC **BREATHS** criteria are absent, no D-dimer

Wells Criteria (Pulmonary Embolism)

Variable	Points
Clinical signs and symptoms of DVT	3
Previous PE or DVT	1.5
Malignancy w/treatment within 6 months or palliative	1
Hemoptysis	1
HR >100 bpm	1.5
PE is #1 diagnosis or equally likely	3
Immobilization at least 3 days or surgery within previous 4 weeks	1.5

Score	Category
1–1.5 points	Low probability
2–6 points	Intermediate probability
6.5 and above points	High probability

Adapted from: Wells PS, Anderson DR, Rodger M, Stiell I, Dreyer JF, Barnes D, Forgie M, Kovacs G, Ward J, Kovacs MJ. Excluding pulmonary embolism at the bedside without diagnostic imaging: management of patients with suspected pulmonary embolism presenting to the emergency department by using a simple clinical model and d-dimer. *Ann Intern Med* 135(2):98–107. (2001)

COPD

Hospital Admission Criteria

- Marked ↑ intensity of sx
- Severe underlying COPD (FEV1 <50 % predicted or on home O_2)
- New signs of cyanosis, edema
- Failure to respond to tx
- Comorbidities, new arrhythmias
- Frequent exacerbations
- Diagnostic uncertainty
- Insufficient home support

ICU Admission Criteria

- Severe dyspnea that inadequately responds to initial ED tx
- Changes in mental status
- Persistent or worsening hypoxia (PaO_2 <40), hypercapnia ($PaCO_2$ >60), or acidosis (pH <7.25) despite treatment
- Need for mechanical ventilation
- Hemodynamically unstable (on vasopressors)

5

Fluid and Electrolytes

B. Allen et al., *Quick Hits in Emergency Medicine,*
DOI 10.1007/978-1-4614-7037-3_5,
© Springer Science+Business Media New York 2013

Hyperkalemia

- Hyper-K? Check EKG
- Wide QRS >100 ms (most sensitive)
  - → Give Ca++
- Tx:
  - Insulin + glucose
  - Beta-agonist
  - Bicarbonate (only if acidotic)
  - Ion exchange resin (controversial due to bowel necrosis)
- 5 ECG changes:
  - Peaked T
  - Prolonged P-R interval
  - Lost P waves
  - Wide QRS >100 ms
  - Sine wave

- Quick Hits for etiology of Hyper-K
  - Not Hyper-K (repeat it!)
  - CRF
  - Acidosis
  - Drugs (ACE+ARB, K-sparing diuretic, NSAIDs, Cox-2 inhibitors)
  - Cell death
    - Tumor lysis (hematologic malignancy?)
    - Rhabdomyolysis or crush injury
    - Burn
    - Hemolysis

Hypokalemia

- Hypo-K? Likely Hypomag Watch for prolonged Q-T!
- Quick Hits for etiology of Hypo-K:
  - Diuretics (thiazides/ furosemide)
  - Malnutrition
  - EtOH
  - Laxative abuse
  - Vomiting

- ECG changes to look for: loss of T waves, U waves, prolonged QTc, Torsades-VT-VF, diffuse ST changes

- Key facts:
  - Usually asymptomatic
  - Repletion takes more than you think
  - 10–20 meq/h PIV is safe
  - Use PO too
  - 10 meq KCl increases K by 0.1 mmol/dL

Hyponatremia

- Usually stable
- Most common cause: diuretic use and low-salt diet
- Give hypertonic saline to a seizing hyponatremic patient
- But remember normal saline is hypertonic relative to patient's hyponatremia
- Correct at 0.5 meq/h or less… NEVER more than 10–12 meq/day

- Only give hypertonic saline:
  - Seizures, acute coma, new focal findings
  - Serum Na 100–110 (always <120)
  - 3 % hypertonic saline

Hyponatremia

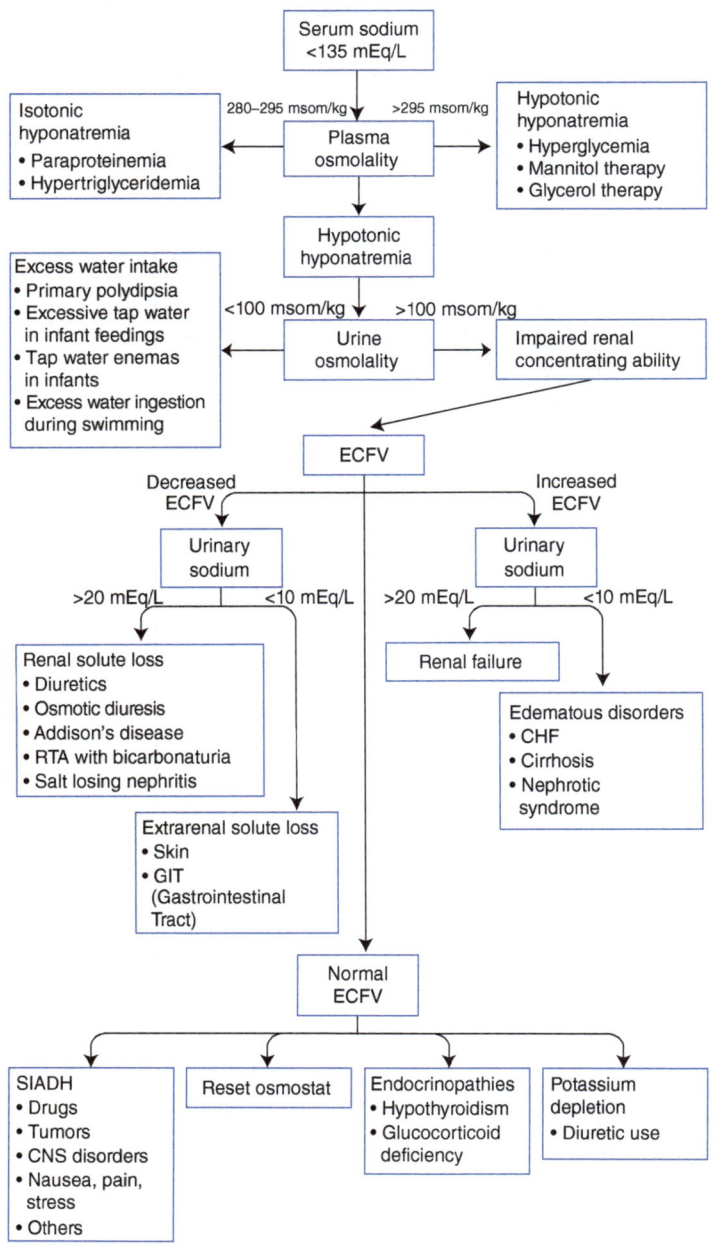

Hypernatremia

- Hypernatremia? Think dehydration and water deficit
- Give fluids, but…
  - Correct slowly!

- Things to keep in mind:
  - Usually geriatric disease
  - Common with AMS
  - Increases mortality for coexisting disease
  - Rapid correction increases mortality

$$\text{Water deficit (liters)} = 0.6 \times (\text{Wt in kg}) \times \left[(Na/140) - 1 \right]$$

Hypercalcemia

- Mild and asymptomatic:
  - Thiazides
  - Other meds
  - Mild overdiuresis
- Severe but asymptomatic:
  - Think hyperparathyroid
- Symptomatic:
  - Think malignancy and paraneoplastic syndrome

- Hypercalcemia? Give saline
- Tx:
  - ABC's
  - Saline (follow I/O)
  - Lasix (forced diuresis)
  - Follow K and Mag
  - Mnemonic: "**PAM P SCHMIDT**"
    - hyper**P**arathyroidism
    - **A**ddison's disease
    - **M**ilk-alkali syndrome
    - **P**aget's disease
    - **S**arcoidosis
    - **C**ancer (paraneoplastic)
    - **H**yperthyroidism
    - **M**yeloma
    - **I**mmobilization
    - **D** (vitamin)
    - **T**hiazides

$$\text{Calcium} = 4 - \text{serum albumin} (g/dL) \times 0.8 + \text{serum calcium}$$

Electrolyte Equations

$$FeNa = \frac{\text{Urine Na/Urine Cr}}{\text{Serum Na/Serum Cr}}$$

* FeNa < 1 → Prerenal

* FeNa > 2 → Intrinsic Renal

Serum Osmolarity:

2Na + BUN/2.8 + Glucose/18 + ETOH/4.6

Spot Urine Na < 20 = likely dehydration

6

Neurology

B. Allen et al., *Quick Hits in Emergency Medicine*,
DOI 10.1007/978-1-4614-7037-3_6,
© Springer Science+Business Media New York 2013

CSF Analysis

	Normal	Preterm term child	Bacterial	Viral	Fungal	TB	Abscess
WBC	0–5	0–25 / 7.3 ± 13.9 / 0–7	>1,000	<1,000	100–500	100–500	10–1,000
% PMN	0–15	57 / 61–84 / 5	>80	<50	<50	<50	<50
% Lymph	>50		<50	>50	>80	Inc. mono	Varies
Glucose	45–65	24–63 / 51.2 ± 12.9 / 40–80	<40	45–65	30–45	30–45	45–60
Ratio	0.6		<0.4	0.6	<0.4	<0.4	0.6
Protein	20–45	65–120 / 64.2 ± 24.2 / 5–40	>150	50–100	100–500	100–500	>50
Pressure	6–20	8–11 / <20 / <20	>25–30	Variable	>20	>20	Variable

San Francisco Syncope Rule

Serious outcome at 7 days is more likely if ANY of the following are present

Hx of CHF

Hct <30

EKG abnormalities (vague)

Shortness of breath/dyspnea

SBP <90

Further workup and/or admission MAY be indicated if any of these high-risk features are present

Adapted from Quinn J, McDermott D, Stiell I, Kohn M, Wells G (May 2006) Prospective validation of the San Francisco Syncope Rule to predict patients with serious outcomes. Ann Emerg Med 47 (5): 448–54

TPA for Stroke

- 0.9 mg/kg over 90 min with 10 % of dose as a bolus over 1 min
- Admit to ICU or stroke unit
- BP and Neuro checks q15 min × 2 h

    – Then q30 min for next 6 h
    – Then q hour for total of 24 h

- Avoid NG tube, Foley and A-line
- Repeat CT scan in 24 h
- *If nausea, vomiting, severe HA, and severe BP elevation occur – STOP infusion and get emergent non-contrast head CT

Adapted from Adams, Harold P. et al. Guidelines for the Early Management of Adults With Ischemic Stroke: A Guideline From the American Heart Association Stroke Council. Stroke May 2007

Stroke and Headache

Stroke Mimics (C²H²AOS)

- **C**onversion disorder
- **C**omplicated migraine
- **H**ypoglycemia
- **H**ypertensive Encephalopathy
- **A**ortic dissection
- **O**ld CVA deficits
- **S**eizure

List is not all-inclusive

Can't Miss HA (PAC³TS)

- **P**seudotumor cerebri
- **A**cute angle closure glaucoma
- **C**ervical artery dissection
- **C**erebral venous thrombosis
- **C**O poisoning
- **T**emporal arteritis
- **S**AH

From Stead et al. First Aid for Emergency Medicine, 3rd Ed.

Vertigo

"SPINNED"	Peripheral vertigo	Central vertigo
Sudden (onset)	Yes	Slow, gradual
Positional	Yes	No
Intensity	Severe	Ill defined
Nausea/diaphoresis	Frequent	Infrequent
Nystagmus	Horizontal	Vertical
Ear (hearing loss)	Can be present	Absent
Duration	Paroxysmal	Constant
CNS signs	Absent	Usually present

7

Trauma and ATLS

B. Allen et al., *Quick Hits in Emergency Medicine,*
DOI 10.1007/978-1-4614-7037-3_7,
© Springer Science+Business Media New York 2013

ATLS Primary Survey

- **A: Airway**
  - Can pt. talk? Voice normal?
  - Stridor? Gag reflex? Foreign body?
  - Bleeding/secretions?
  - Burns?
- **B: Breathing**
  - Equal chest rise/fall?
  - Breath sounds bilat.? SQ air?
  - Deviated trachea? JVD? Flail chest/fracture?
- **C: Circulation**
  - Heart sounds, pulses in all ext.
  - Look for external bleeding
  - Get vascular access
- **D: Disability**
  - Alert, verbal, painful stimuli, unresponsive (AVPU)
  - GCS, gross motor/sensory, pupils
- **E:** Exposure (get all clothes off)

- **F:** Finger
  - Rectal exam (controversial but still ATLS)
- **F:** FAST
  - Looking for hemoperitoneum and/or pericardial effusion
- **F:** Foley
  - Contraindicated for blood at meatus and high-riding prostate
- **F:** Family
  - Notify next of kin ASAP
- **F:** Fentanyl
  - Appropriate pain control
  - Fentanyl most hemodynamically stable narcotic
  - Prevent hypothermia

Adapted from Sanjay Arora "Trauma Review 2009" USC Essentials 2009

ATLS History

"AMPLE-F"

A	Allergies
M	Medications
P	PMH
L	Last meal/LMP
E	Events of trauma (what happened)
F	Family, friends, field personnel

Adapted from Sanjay Arora "Trauma Review 2009" USC Essentials 2009

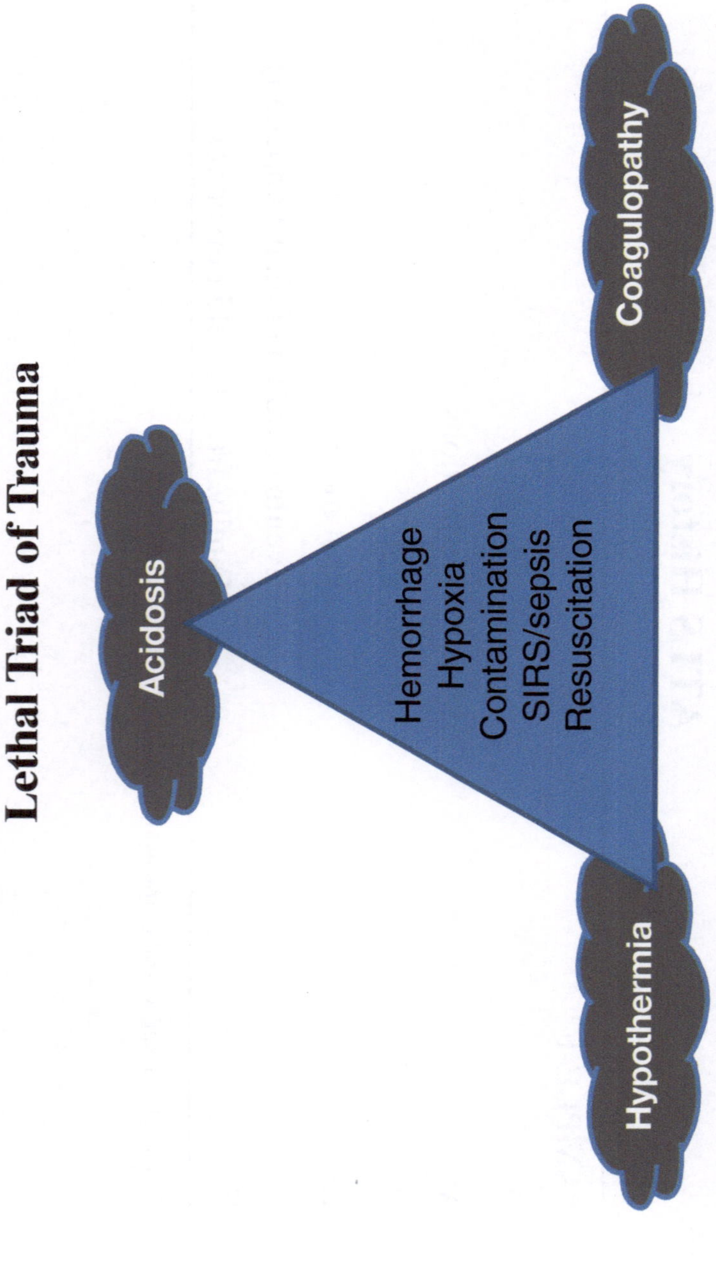

Lethal Triad of Trauma

Acidosis

Coagulopathy

Hypothermia

Hemorrhage
Hypoxia
Contamination
SIRS/sepsis
Resuscitation

GCS

Eye opening	Best verbal	Best motor
4 – Spontaneous	5 – Oriented/converses	6 – Obeys
3 – Verbal command	4 – Disoriented/converses	5 – Localizes pain
2 – Pain	3 – Inappropriate words	4 – Withdraw to stim
1 – No response	2 – Incomprehensible	3 – Abn flex/decort
	1 – No response	2 – Abn ext/decer
		1 – No response

Trauma Checklist

- Hgb (serial)
- Initial and repeat VS
- FAST (serial)
- External bleeders controlled?
- Labs sent (type screen/cross?)
- Airway secured (present/future)

- Life/limb threats addressed
- Spine immobilized
- Large bore access × 2
- Pain meds
- "AMPLE-F" history comorbidities?

Shock in Trauma

Type of shock	Physical findings/clues
Hemorrhagic shock (hypovolemic shock)	Narrow pulse pressure, external bleeding, flat neck veins
Tension pneumothorax (obstructive shock)	Absent unilateral breath sounds, deviated trachea, JVD, narrow pulse pressure, pulsus paradoxus
Cardiac tamponade (obstructive shock)	JVD, muffled heart sounds, narrow pulse pressure, pulsus paradoxus
Myocardial contusion (cardiogenic shock)	Persistent tachycardia, abnormal ECG, and/or cardiac enzymes
Neurogenic shock	Hypotension and bradycardia, warm extremities, injury above T6

Hemorrhage Classifications

	Class I	Class II	Class III	Class IV
Blood loss (ml)	≤750	750–1,500	1,500–2,000	≥2,000
Blood loss (% bold volume)	≤15	15–30	30–40	≥40
Pulse rate (per min)	<100	>100	>120	≥140
Blood pressure	Normal	Normal	Decreased	Decreased
Pulse pressure	Normal or increased	Decreased	Decreased	Decreased
Capillary refill test	Normal	Positive	Positive	Positive
Respiratory rate (breaths · min^{-1})	14–20	20–30	30–40	<35
Urine output (ml · h^{-1})	≥30	20–30	5–15	Negligible
CNS mental status	Slightly anxious	Mildly anxious	Anxious and confused	Confused, lethargic
Fluid replacement (3:1 rule)	Crystalloid	Crystalloid	Crystalloid + blood	Crystalloid + blood

Burn Classifications

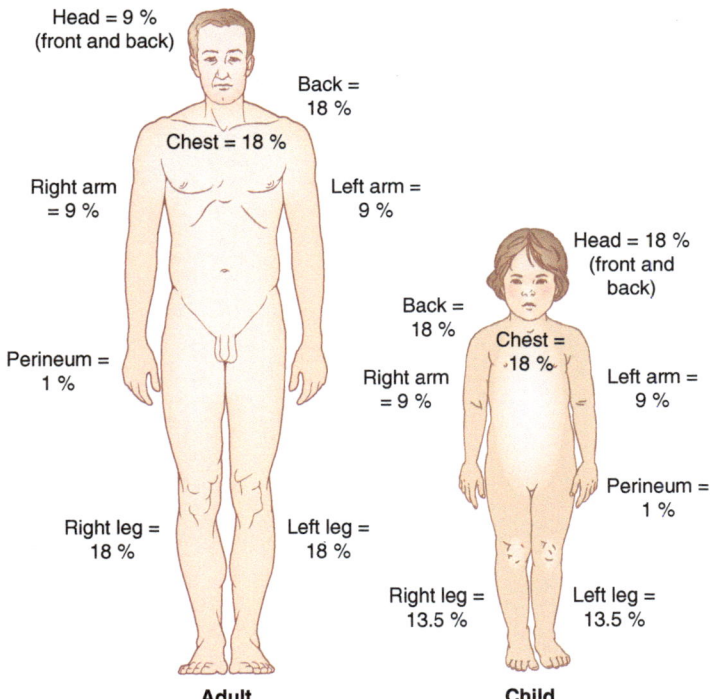

Head = 9 %
(front and back)

Back =
18 %

Chest = 18 %

Right arm
= 9 %

Left arm =
9 %

Perineum =
1 %

Right leg =
18 %

Left leg =
18 %

Adult

Head = 18 %
(front and
back)

Back =
18 %

Chest =
18 %

Right arm
= 9 %

Left arm =
9 %

Perineum =
1 %

Right leg =
13.5 %

Left leg =
13.5 %

Child

Parkland Formula = LR 4ml/kg/% burn TBSA in
first 24 h + maintain fluids w/half in first 8 h + second half in last 16 h

8

Head CT Decision Rules and Intracranial Hemorrhage

B. Allen et al., *Quick Hits in Emergency Medicine*,
DOI 10.1007/978-1-4614-7037-3_8,
© Springer Science+Business Media New York 2013

Mild Head Injury/TBI

- Can be direct impact to skull or brain that results in disturbance of brain function (think falls, syncope, MVC, assault)
- Do not underestimate prevalence or associated morbidity
- 25 % of GCS 15 head trauma will have abnormal CT
- LOC, AOC, PTA, and Sz all associated with worse TBI severity and outcomes
- 25 % develop post-concussive syndrome (sleep difficulties, fatigue, irritability, poor concentration, headache)
- Patients on anticoagulants have higher risk of poor outcome
- No single best way to diagnose—CT, MRI, EEG, neurocognitive tests—none perfect
- Image, check vision, rx antiemetic, and non-opiate analgesia provide f/u
- Most important instruction is complete brain rest for 5–7 days:
  <1 h screen time per day: includes texting, video games, TV Rest in a low-stimulation environment: no bright lights, no loud sounds GRADUAL return to daily activities

Nexus-II Head CT Decision Rule

- Nexus-II (100 % sensitivity)
  1. Altered (AMS)
  2. Suspicion of fracture
  3. Current vomiting
  4. Age >65
  5. Neurologic deficits
  6. Coagulopathy
  7. Scalp hematoma
     - LOC is not absolute indication for Head CT
     - Valid for immediate presentation only

Adapted from: Mower et al. NEXUS II (the National Emergency X-Radiography Utilization Study: J Trauma 2005;59[4]:954; Ann Emerg Med 2002;40[5]:505)

Canadian Head CT Decision Rule

High-risk features predictive of need for neurosurgical intervention

- GCS <15 at 2 h after injury
- Suspected open or depressed skull fracture
- Signs of basal skull fracture
- At least 2 episodes of vomiting
- Age ≥65 years old

Medium-risk features for brain injury detection on CT

- Amnesia before impact of ≥30 min
- Dangerous mechanism (pedestrian vs auto, an occupant ejected from a motor vehicle, or a fall from an elevation of ≥3 ft or 5 stairs)

→ **CT indicated if any of the above are present**

Adapted from: Stiell IG, Wells GA, Vandemheen K, Clement C, Lesiuk H, Laupacis A, McKnight RD, Verbeek R, Brison R, Cass D, Eisenhauer ME, Greenberg G, Worthington J. The Canadian CT Head Rule for patients with minor head injury. Lancet. 2001 May 5;357(9266):1391–6

New Orleans Criteria

Head CT Decision Rule

1. HA
2. Vomiting
3. Age >60
4. Intoxication
5. Persistent anterograde amnesia
6. Trauma above clavicles
7. Seizure

Presence of any = head CT

- Stats and caveats:
  - 100 % sens and 5 % spec for both requiring surgery and for any intracranial lesion
  - Can't apply to peds or pts on anticoagulants

Adapted from: Haydel MJ, Preston CA, Mills TJ, Luber S, Blaudeau E, DeBlieux PM. Indications for computed tomography in patients with minor head injury. N Engl J Med. 2000 Jul 13;343(2):100–5.

Reading a Head CT

- Blood Can Be Very Bad
- B: Blood (look for blood): subdural, Epi, SAH
- C: Cisterns
  - Key view #1: basal cistern at level of pons
  - Key view #2: quadrigeminal cisterns (frown = bad)
- B: Brain (look for asymmetry)
  - Diffuse axonal injury, SAH, nontraumatic lesions, contusions
- V: Ventricles
  - Blood?
- B: Bone
  - Look for fx or air adjacent to bone
  - Hemotympanum on exam? Look for mastoid fx

Epidural Hematoma

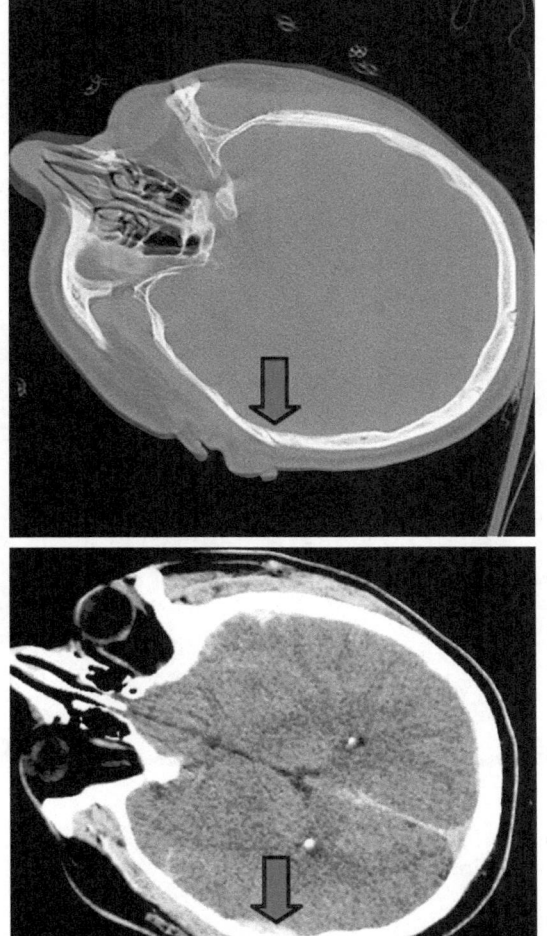

Used with permission from Stead et al., First Aid for the Radiology Clerkship, McGraw Hill

Subdural Hematoma

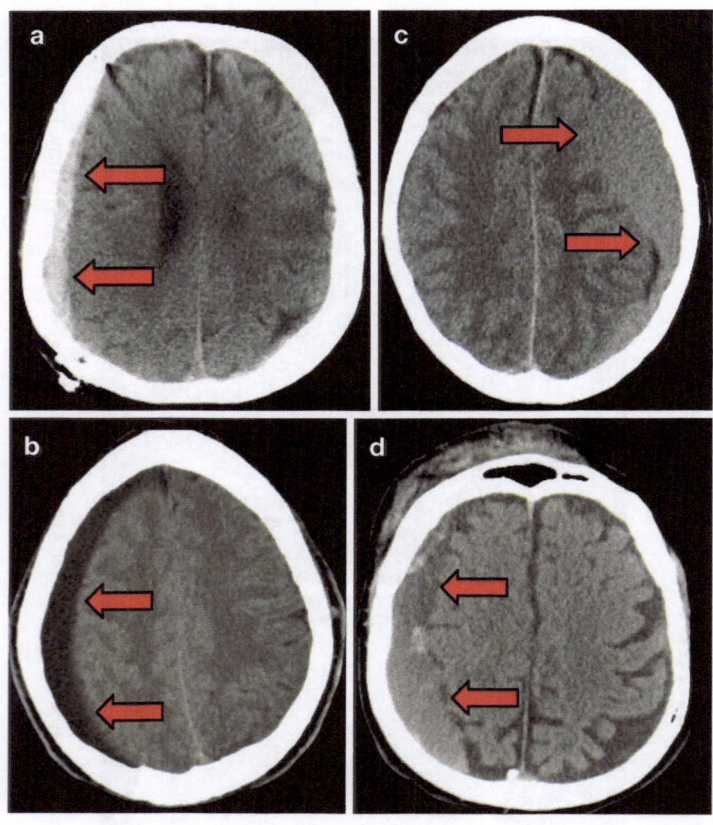

Used with permission from Stead et al., First Aid for the Radiology Clerkship, McGraw Hill

Subarachnoid Hemorrhage

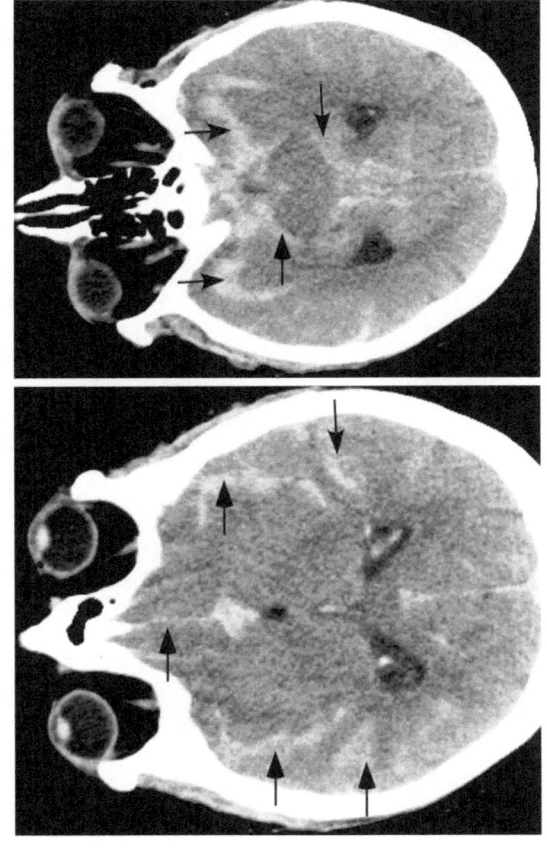

9

Cervical Spine Injury and Decision Rules

B. Allen et al., *Quick Hits in Emergency Medicine*,
DOI 10.1007/978-1-4614-7037-3_9,
© Springer Science+Business Media New York 2013

Cervical Spine Alignment and Allowable Distances

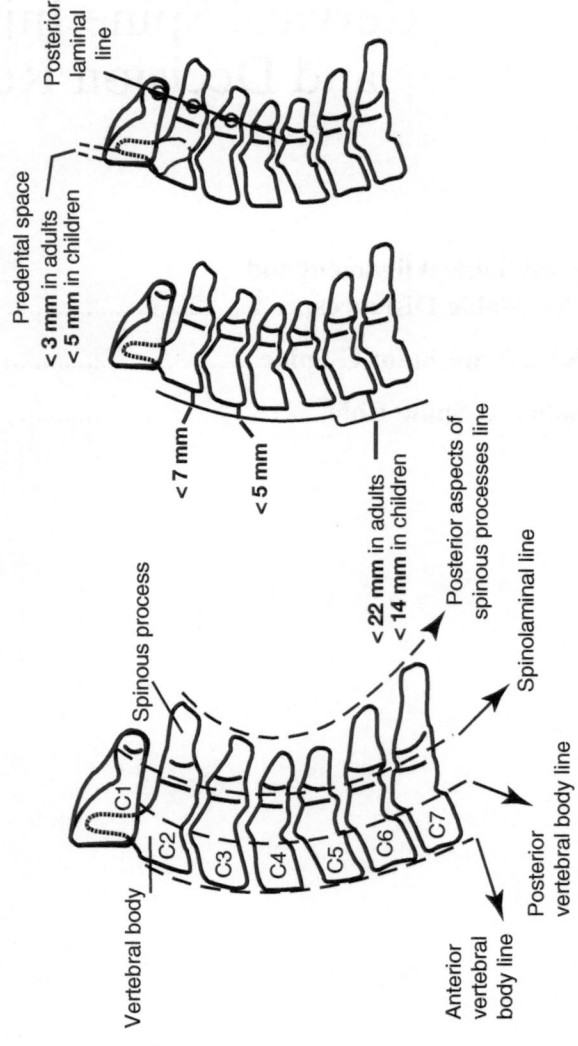

Used with permission from First aid for emergency medicine clerkship by Stead et al., McGraw Hill

NEXUS Criteria for C-Spine

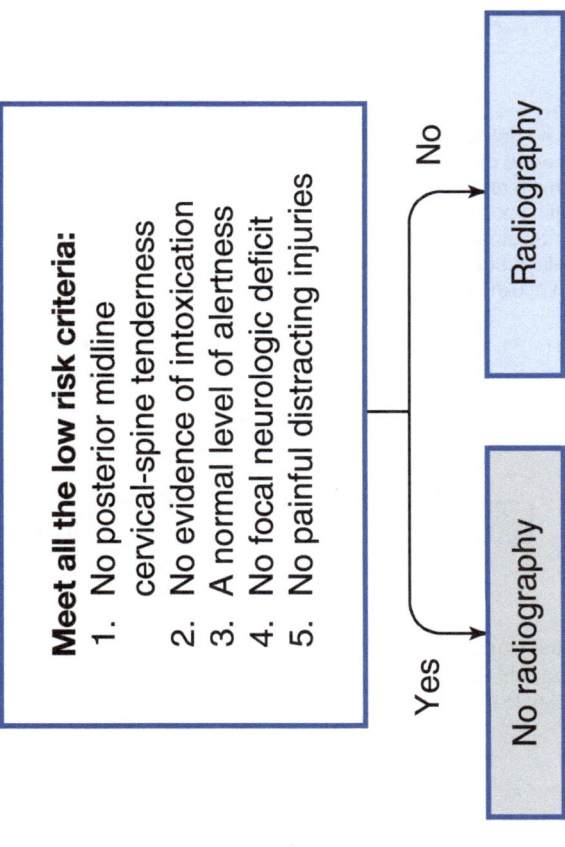

Meet all the low risk criteria:

1. No posterior midline cervical-spine tenderness
2. No evidence of intoxication
3. A normal level of alertness
4. No focal neurologic deficit
5. No painful distracting injuries

Yes → No radiography

No → Radiography

Adapted from: Hoffman JR, Wolfson AB, Todd K, Mower WR. Selective cervical spine radiography in blunt trauma: methodology of the National Emergency X-Radiography Utilization Study (NEXUS). Ann Emerg Med. 1998 Oct;32(4):461–9

Canadian C-Spine Rule

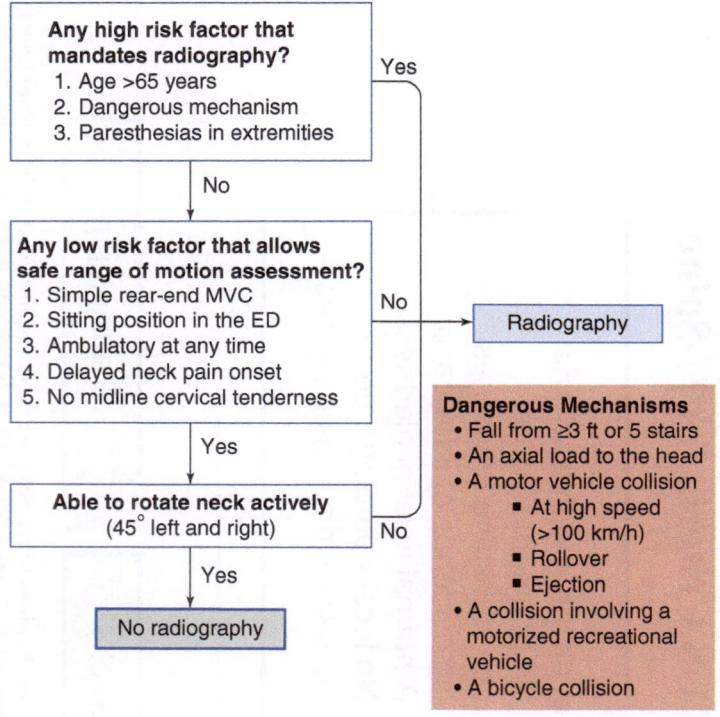

Adapted from: Stiell IG, Wells GA, Vandemheen KL, et al. The Canadian C-spine rule for radiography in alert and stable trauma patients. JAMA. 2001;286(15):1841–1848

CXR Interpretation

B. Allen et al., *Quick Hits in Emergency Medicine*,
DOI 10.1007/978-1-4614-7037-3_10,
© Springer Science+Business Media New York 2013

CXR Interpretation

- Organized approach
- Outside the chest
- Soft tissues, bones, abdomen
- Chest
- Diaphragms, airway, aorta, + mediastinum, pericardium and heart, pleura and lungs

- Pneumothorax in trauma: look for deep sulcus sign and sharp diaphragm or double diaphragm (often missed)

CXR Interpretation

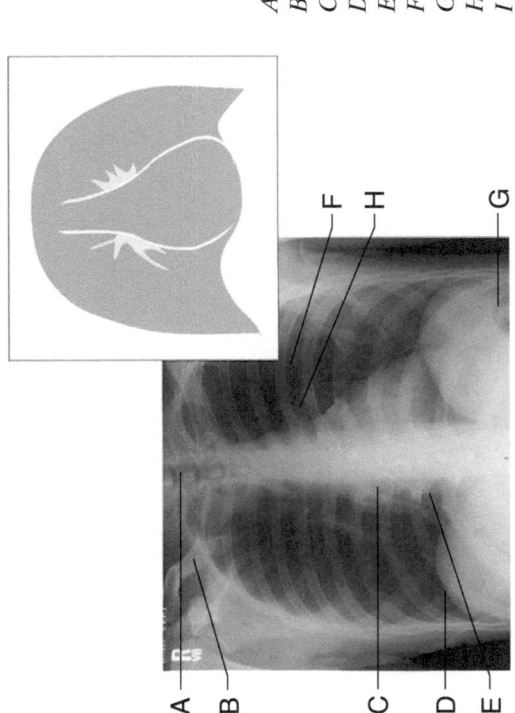

A Airway,
B Bones,
C Cardiac silhouette/size,
D Diaphragm,
E Edges (Heart borders),
F Fields (Lungs),
G Gastric bubble,
H Hilum,
I Instrumentation (Tubes and lines)

11

Orthopedics and Decision Rules

B. Allen et al., *Quick Hits in Emergency Medicine*,
DOI 10.1007/978-1-4614-7037-3_11,
© Springer Science+Business Media New York 2013

Ottawa Ankle and Foot Rules

X-rays are required only if there is bony pain over the malleolar or midfoot area and any one of the following:

Bone tenderness along the distal 6 cm of the posterior edge of the tibia or tip of the medial malleolus

Bone tenderness along the distal 6 cm of the posterior edge of the fibula or tip of the lateral malleolus

Bone tenderness at the base of the fifth metatarsal (foot injuries and concern for Jones fracture)

Bone tenderness at the navicular bone (foot injury)

Inability to bear weight both immediately after the injury and for 4 steps in the ED (within 10 days of injury)

Adapted from Stiell IG, McKnight RD, Greenberg GH, et al.: Implementation of the Ottawa Rules. JAMA 271:827, 1994

Ottawa Knee Rules

Knee X-rays are indicated if ANY of the following are present (97–100 % sens for fracture)

Age ≥55

Pain at the head of the fibula

Isolated patella tenderness

Can't flex knee 90°

Inability to walk 4 weight-bearing steps BOTH immediately AND in ED (regardless of limp)

Adapted from Stiell IG, Wells GA, Hoag RH, et al.: Implementation of the Ottawa Knee Rules for the use of radiography in acute knee injuries. JAMA 278:2075, 1997

Orthopedics

Compartment Syndrome

- 6 P's:
  - Pain
  - Pallor
  - Paresthesia
  - Pulselessness (late)
  - Poikilothermia
  - Paralysis

- Delta P:
  - Diastolic BP-compartment
  - Delta $P < 30$ = Fasciotomy

Flexor Tenosynovitis

- Kanavel's 4 signs:
  - Fusiform swelling
  - Flexed position
  - Pain with passive flexion/extension
  - Proximal tenderness along the tendon sheath

Orthopedic Disposition

ORTHO NOW
- Neurovascular compromise and compartment sx
- Open fracture or non-reduced dislocations
- Severe infx (necrotizing fasciitis, flexor tenosynovitis, closed space infx, abscess, post-op infx)
- "Major Ortho Trauma" (pelvic, femur, tibial plateau, tibial shaft)
- Amputations (depends on location)

ORTHO Follow-up
- Fracture likely requiring surgery (ankle, wrist, elbow, prox. humerus, etc.)
  - Severe comminution or intra-articular
- Tendon laceration/rupture
- Infection follow-ups (48–72 h)

12

Cardiology

B. Allen et al., *Quick Hits in Emergency Medicine*,
DOI 10.1007/978-1-4614-7037-3_12,
© Springer Science+Business Media New York 2013

Differential Diagnosis of Chest Pain

Life-threatening causes of chest pain	Non-life-threatening causes of chest pain
Acute coronary syndrome (ACS)	Pericarditis
Esophageal rupture	Esophageal spasm
Pericardial tamponade	Esophageal reflux (GERD)
Pneumothorax	Chest wall pain
Pulmonary embolism	Pleurisy
	Peptic ulcer disease (PUD)
	Biliary disease
	Panic attack (anxiety disorder)
	Cervical arthritis (radiculopathy)

Acute Coronary Syndrome

- Indicators of acute MI
  - 1 mm or more ST segment elevation in 2 contiguous leads
  - Reciprocal ST depression
  - Q waves
  - Always compare to old ECG's
  - Repeat ECG in 15–30 min

1. Atypical is typical—atypical CP doesn't r/o MI
2. Beware the geriatric patient with atypical symptoms
3. Delta enzyme analysis
4. Use objective test or provocative study

STEMI vs Benign Early Repolarization (BER)

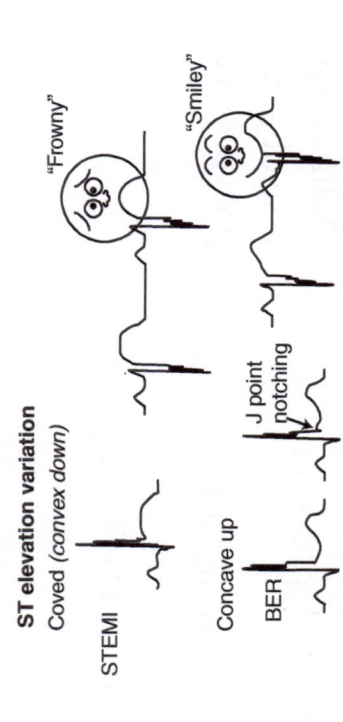

ST elevation variation

Coved (*convex down*)

"Frowny"

STEMI

"Smiley"

Concave up

BER

J point notching

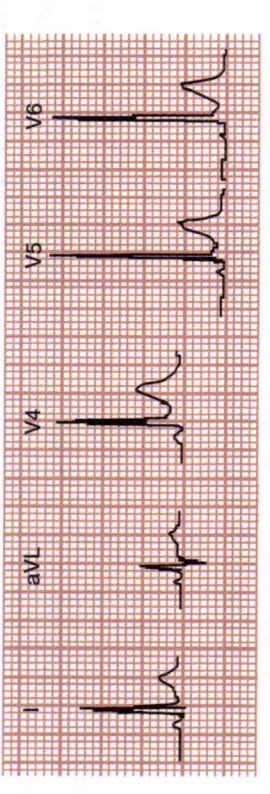

I   aVL   V4   V5   V6

Left Ventricular Hypertrophy (LVH)

- S in V1 + R in V5 or V6 > 35 mm *or*

  − S in V1 *or* V2 + R in V5 or V6 > 35 mm

- R in aVL > 11 mm
- R in V4–6 > 25mm
- S in V1–3 > 25 mm
- R in I + S in III > 25 mm

New Onset A-fib

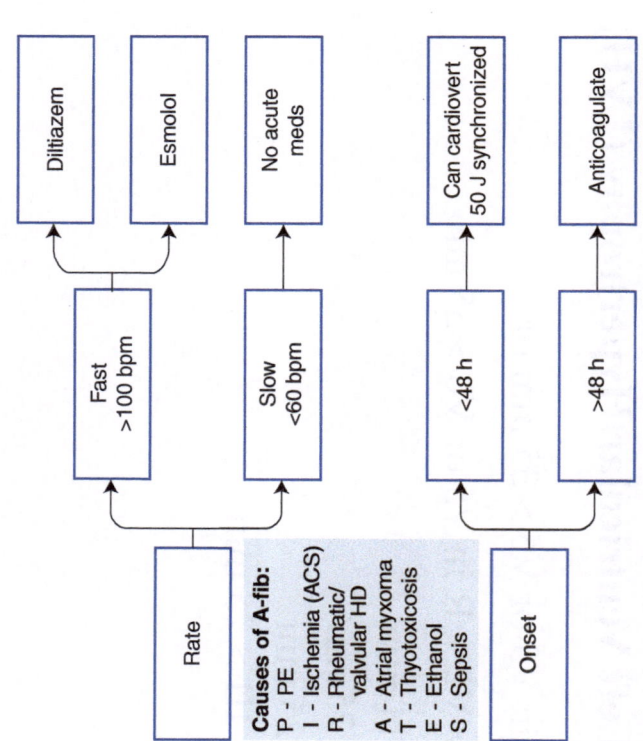

Diltiazem

Esmolol

No acute meds

Can cardiovert 50 J synchronized

Anticoagulate

Fast >100 bpm

Slow <60 bpm

<48 h

>48 h

Rate

Onset

Causes of A-fib:
P - PE
I - Ischemia (ACS)
R - Rheumatic/ valvular HD
A - Atrial myxoma
T - Thyotoxicosis
E - Ethanol
S - Sepsis

Left Atrial Hypertrophy (LAH)

- Notched P wave with >40 ms between the two peaks with total P wave duration >110 ms
- **In V1**
  - Biphasic P wave with terminal negative portion >40 ms duration
  - Biphasic P wave with terminal negative portion >1 mm deep

Sgarbossa's Criteria

Diagnosis of acute MI in the presence of left bundle branch block (LBBB)

Criteria for diagnosis of acute MI (Sgarbossa's criteria)	POINTS
ST elevation >1 mm concordant (same direction) as QRS	5
ST depression >1 mm in leads V1, V2, or V3	3
ST elevation >5 mm and discordant (opposite) with QRS	2
Total >3 is 36–78 % sensitive, 90–96 % specific for acute MI	

Adapted from Elena. B. Sgarbossa et al.; New England Journal of Medicine, Volume 334; Number 8, Feb 22, 1996

Sgarbossa's Criteria

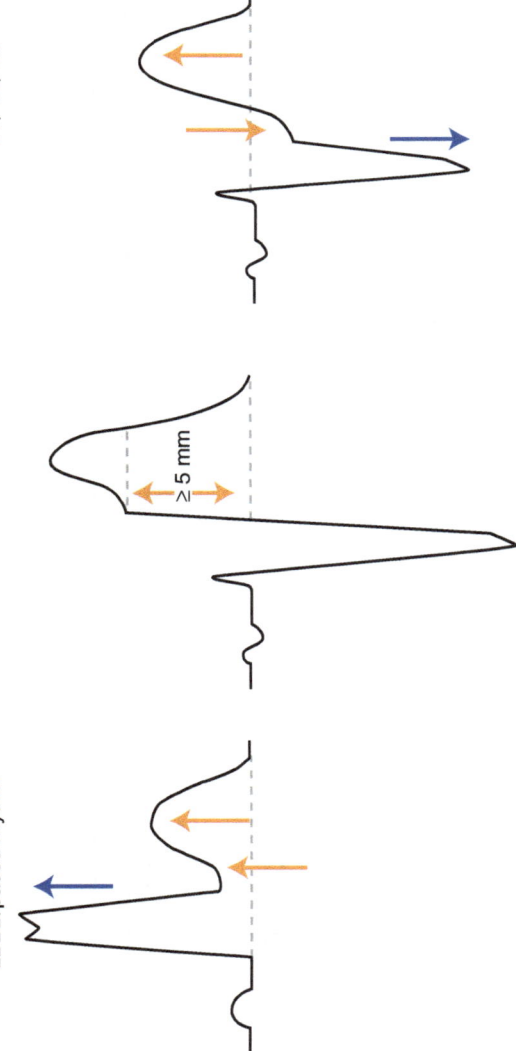

Brugada Syndrome

Diagnostic criteria for Brugada syndrome ST-segment abnormalities in leads V1–V3

	Type 1	Type 2	Type 3
J-point	≥2 mm	≥2 mm	≥2 mm
T wave	Negative	Positive or biphasic	Positive
ST-T configuration	Coved type	Saddleback	Saddleback
ST segment (terminal portion)	Gradually descending	Elevated ≥1 mm	Elevated <1 mm

1 mm = 0.1 mV; the terminal portion of the ST segment refers to the latter half of the ST segment (From Wilde et al. with permission)

Brugada Criteria for V-Tach

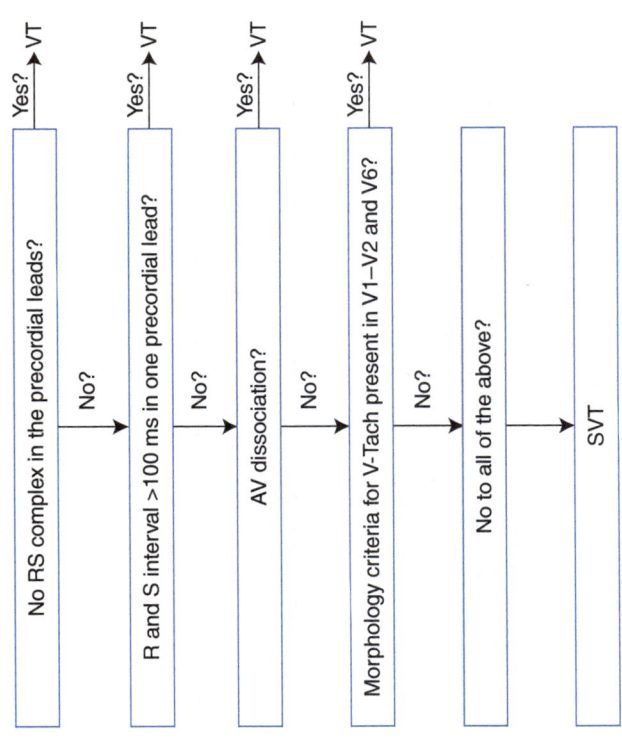

No RS complex in the precordial leads? — Yes? → VT
No? ↓

R and S interval >100 ms in one precordial lead? — Yes? → VT
No? ↓

AV dissociation? — Yes? → VT
No? ↓

Morphology criteria for V-Tach present in V1–V2 and V6? — Yes? → VT
No? ↓

No to all of the above?
↓

SVT

Wellens' Sign/Syndrome

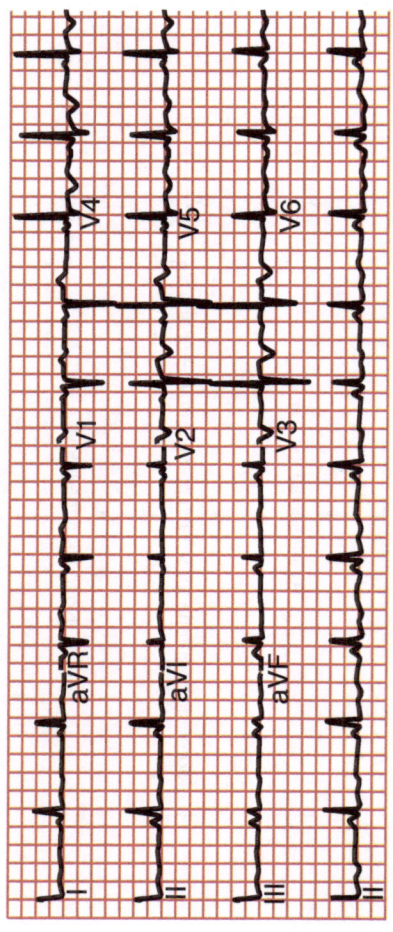

Criteria of Wellens' Syndrome

- Prior history of chest pain
- Chest pain with normal ECG
- Normal or minimally elevated cardiac enzymes
- No pathologic precordial Q waves or loss of R waves
- St segment in V2 and V3 that is isoelectric or minimally elevated (1 mm), concave, or straight
- Symmetric and deep T wave inversion or byphasic T waves in V2–V5 or V6 in pain free periods
- Tight proximal LAD stenosis

13

GI Bleeding/Hemorrhage

B. Allen et al., *Quick Hits in Emergency Medicine,*
DOI 10.1007/978-1-4614-7037-3_13,
© Springer Science+Business Media New York 2013

GI Bleeding/Hemorrhage

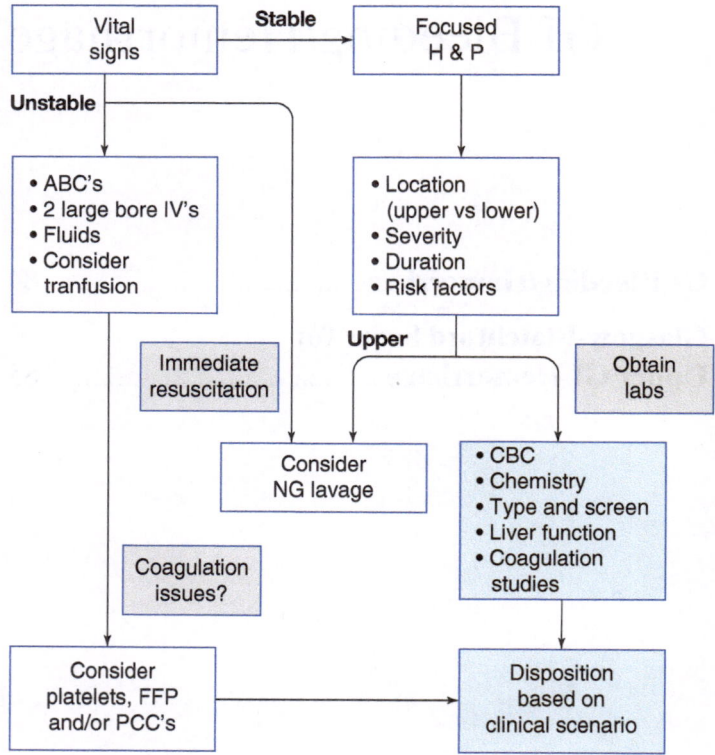

Glasgow-Blatchford Score for Upper GI Hemorrhage

A score of zero and Pt is low risk for serious outcome if all below are present:

Hgb >12.9 (men) or >11.9 (women)

SBP >109 mmHg

HR <100 bpm

BUN <18.2 mg/dL

No melena

No syncope

No past or present liver disease

No past or present heart failure

Stanley A, Ashley D, Dalton H, et al. Outpatient management of patients with low-risk upper-gastrointestinal haemorrhage: multicentre validation and prospective evaluation. Lancet January 3, 2009;373(9657):42–47

Hematology

B. Allen et al., *Quick Hits in Emergency Medicine,*
DOI 10.1007/978-1-4614-7037-3_14,
© Springer Science+Business Media New York 2013

ITP/TTP/DIC

- Thrombocytopenia? r/o TTP before giving platelets
- MAHA (schistocytes on peripheral smear)? Think TTP!
- TTP needs plasma exchange Transfusion

Mnemonic: "**FAT RN**"

  Fever
  Anemia
  Thrombocytopenia
  Renal (kidney injury)
  Neurologic complaints

	ITP	TTP	DIC
Dec. platelets	Yes	Yes	Yes
Inc. PT/INR	No	No	Yes
MAHA	No	Yes	No
Normal fibrin-fibrinogen	Yes	Yes	No
"Sick"	No	Yes	Yes
Ok to give platelets	Yes if critical	No death	Yes

15

Toxicology

B. Allen et al., *Quick Hits in Emergency Medicine,*
DOI 10.1007/978-1-4614-7037-3_15,
© Springer Science+Business Media New York 2013

Toxidromes

Anticholinergic	Cholinergic
Mydriasis	Salivation
Hypertension	Lacrimation
Decreased bowel sounds	Urination
Tachycardia	Diarrhea/defecation
Skin flushing, dry skin	Emesis
AMS/confusion, agitation/hallucinations	Bradycardia
Urinary retention	Bronchorrhea/bronchospasm
Tx: consider physostigmine	**Tx: decontamination — atropine and pralidoxime (2-PAM)**

Ingestions

Acetaminophen OD

- Always use 4–20 h APAP level to determine risk
  - Consider 8 h level if extended release APAP
- Clinical findings
  - N/V, pallor, malaise
  - Hepatotoxicity after 24 h
  - Depression/suicide (always ask)
- NAC is mainstay of therapy
- Call poison control

ASA OD

- Toxic levels evident at 6 h
  - Wintergreen and bismuth contain ASA
- Initial increased RR (resp alkalosis)
- Primary AG met acidosis
- N/V/tinnitus/sweating
- Acute pulmonary edema
- Toxic dose = 150–200 mg/kg
- Dialysis is the definitive therapy
- Call poison control

Acetaminophen Nomogram

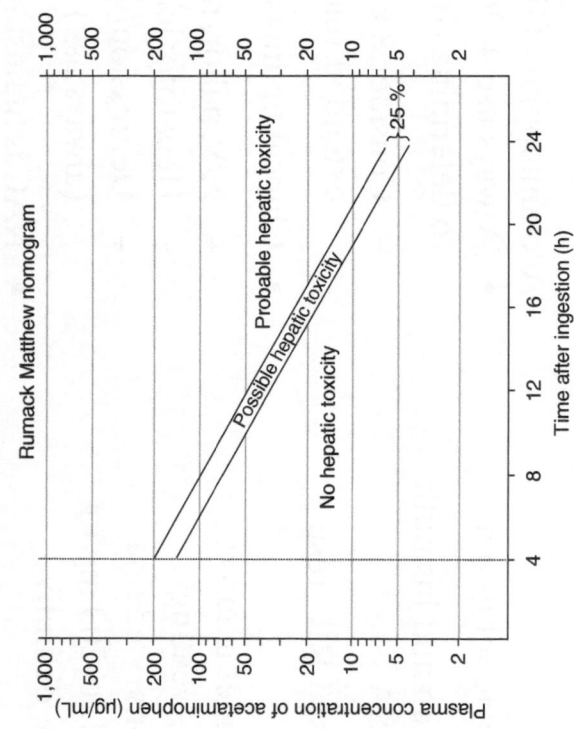

Used with permission from First Aid for the Emergency Medicine Clerkship 3rd Ed., by Stead et al, McGraw Hill, 2011.

Toxicology

Coma Cocktail

- **DON'T**
  - **Dextrose** (1 amp D50)
  - **Oxygen** (supplemental)
  - **Narcan** (titrate slowly)
  - **Thiamine** (to prevent Wernicke's)

Ingestion	Antidote
APAP	NAC
Anticholinergic	Physostigmine
Benzodiazepines	Flumazenil (controversial)
Beta-blockers	Glucagon
Ca channel blockers	Glucagon, Ca, insulin
Cholinergic	Atropine
Digoxin	Digibind
Ethylene glycol	Fomepizole, dialysis
Iron	Deferoxamine
INH	B6 (pyridoxine)
Methanol	Fomepizole, dialysis
Methemoglobinemia	Methylene blue
Organophosphates	Pralidoxime, atropine
Salicylates and TCA	Sodium bicarbonate, dialysis

Toxicology

Non-anion Gap Metabolic Acidosis

- **USED CAR**
  - **U**remia
  - **S**aline
  - **E**nteric fistula
  - **D**iarrhea
  - **C**arbonic anhydrase inhibitors
  - **A**cids (exogenous)
  - **R**enal tubular acidosis

Anion Gap Metabolic Acidosis

- **CAT MUDPILES**
  - **C**arbon monoxide/cyanide
  - **A**lcoholic ketoacidosis
  - **T**oluene
  - **M**ethanol
  - **U**remia
  - **D**KA
  - **P**henothiazines (Haldol)
  - **I**NH
  - **L**actate
  - **E**TOH, ethylene glycol
  - **S**alicylates

Toxicology

Radiopaque Substances

- **CHIPS**
  - **C**hlorinated substances (pesticides)
  - **H**eavy metals (lead, mercury, arsenic)
  - **I**odine/**I**ron
  - **P**henothiazines
  - **S**ustained-release tabs/salicylates (enteric coated)

Dialyzable Toxins

- **I STUMBLE**
  - **I**sopropyl
  - **S**alicylates
  - **T**heophylline
  - **U**remia
  - **M**ethanol
  - **B**arbiturates
  - **L**ithium
  - **E**thylene glycol/ETOH

Serotonin Syndrome

Hunter Serotonin Toxicity Criteria (if serotonergic agent is present)

Diagnosis of serotonin syndrome can be made if at least one of the criteria is present

1. Spontaneous clonus

2. Inducible clonus and agitation or diaphoresis

3. Ocular clonus and agitation or diaphoresis

4. Tremor and hyperreflexia

5. Hypertonicity and fever (>38 C) and ocular clonus or inducible clonus

If none of the above criteria present, not serotonin syndrome/toxicity

Adapted from: Dunkley EJ, Isbister GK, Sibbritt D, Dawson AH, Whyte IM (September 2003). "The Hunter Serotonin Toxicity Criteria: simple and accurate diagnostic decision rules for serotonin toxicity". *QJM* 96 (9): 635–42

Coma "AEIOU TIPS"

A: Alcohol

E: Encephalopathy, endocrine (thyroid, etc.), electrolyte abnormality

I: IDDM

O: Opiates, oxygen deprivation

U: Uremia

T: Trauma, temperature

I: Infection

P: Psychosis, porphyria

S: Space-occupying lesion, stroke, SAH, shock

16

Ultrasound and Pregnancy

B. Allen et al., *Quick Hits in Emergency Medicine,*
DOI 10.1007/978-1-4614-7037-3_16,
© Springer Science+Business Media New York 2013

Ultrasound

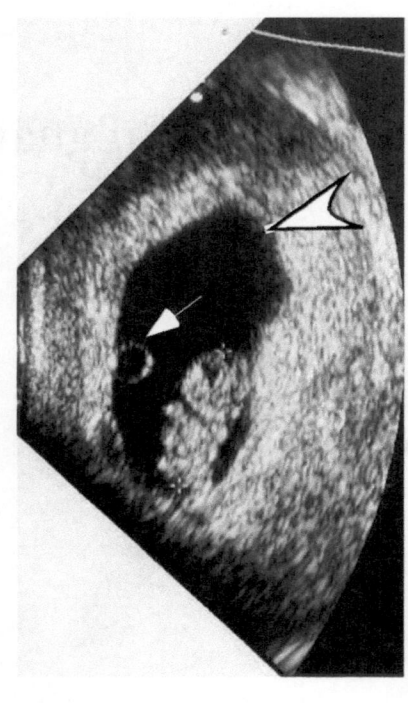

Used with permission from First Aid for the Emergency Medicine Clerkship 3rd Ed., by Stead et al., McGraw Hill, 2011

Transvaginal US IUP Findings

- Gestational sac (arrowhead):
  - HCG >1,000 (5 weeks)
- Yolk sac (arrow):
  - HCG > 2,500
- Heart tones:
  - HCG > 10,500–17,000

Ectopic Pregnancy

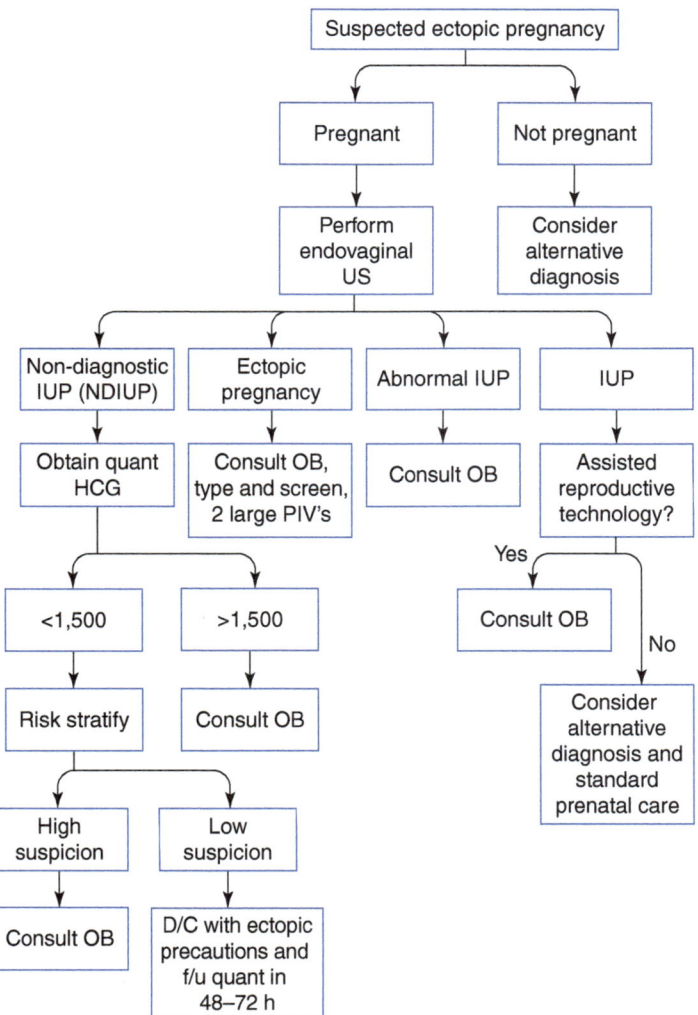

Reproduced with permission of F. E. Flach, M.D. University of Florida Pregnancy Algorithm

17

The Red Eye

B. Allen et al., *Quick Hits in Emergency Medicine*,
DOI 10.1007/978-1-4614-7037-3_17,
© Springer Science+Business Media New York 2013

The Red Eye

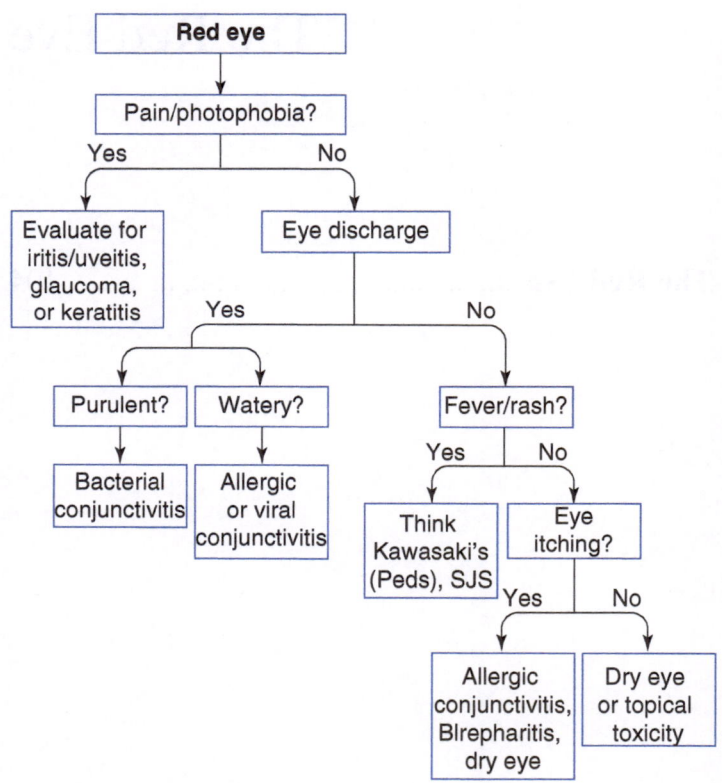

18

Pediatrics

B. Allen et al., *Quick Hits in Emergency Medicine*,
DOI 10.1007/978-1-4614-7037-3_18,
© Springer Science+Business Media New York 2013

Pediatric Vital Signs

Age	RR	HR	SBP	DBP
Neonate (30 days)	40–60	100–180 (195)	60–90	20–60
1–12 months	30–60	100–160 (195)	70–110	50–70
13–24 months	24–40	80–110 (132)	74–110	55–75
2–5 years	22–34	70–110 (132)	80–112	55–75
6–7 years	18–30	65–110 (132)	85–115	57–75
8 (adolescent)	16–20	65–90 (108)	95–125	65–80

HR in parentheses represents possible HR in febrile otherwise healthy child

Kocher Criteria

Criteria

- Erythrocyte sedimentation Rate >40
- WBC >12
- Non-weight-bearing of the lower extremity
- Fever

Scoring

- If only one sign is present, there is a 3 % chance the child has a septic hip
- 2/4 criteria = 40 %
- 3/4 criteria = 93 %
- 4/4 criteria = 99 %

Adapted from Kocher et al. Validation of a Clinical Prediction Rule for the Differentiation Between Septic Arthritis and Transient Synovitis of the Hip in Children. The Journal of Bone and Joint Surgery (American) 86:1629–1635 (2004).

Pediatrics

APGAR

- Appearance
  - 2: Entire body pink
  - 1: Body pink, extremities blue
  - 0: Entire body blue
- Pulse
  - 2: >100
  - 1: <100
  - 0: Absent
- Grimace
  - 2: Vigorous cry, cough, sneeze
  - 1: Grimace, weak cry
  - 0: No response
- Activity
  - 2: Active
  - 1: Some
  - 0: None
- Respirations
  - 2: Strong
  - 1: Weak, irregular
  - 0: None

ETT Size/Depth
- Use Broselow tape!
- Formula uncuffed $= (Age/4) + 4$

Salter-Harris Fractures (SALTR)

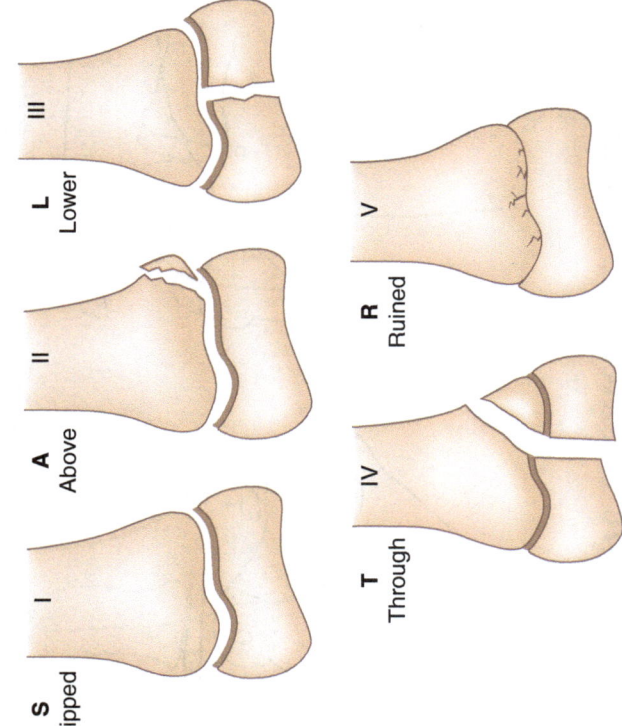

Pediatric Ossification Centers

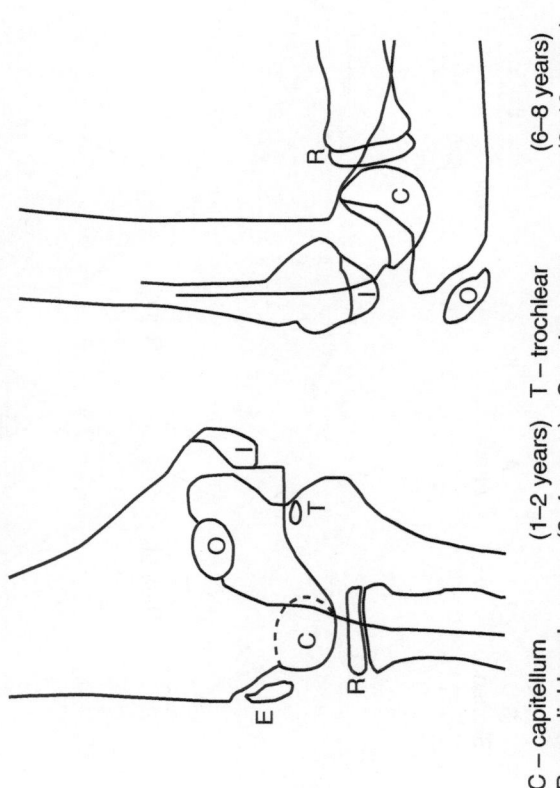

C – capitellum   (1–2 years)   T – trochlear   (6–8 years)
R – radial head   (2–4 years)   O – olecronon   (8–10 years)
I – internal malleous   (4–6 years)   E – external malleolus (10–12 years)

Pediatric GCS

Eye opening	Verbal	Motor
4—Spontaneous	5—Age-appropriate speech	6—Obeys commands or spontaneous movement
3—To voice	4—Less than usual; irritable cry	5—Localizes pain
2—To pain	3—Cries to pain	4—Withdraws pain
1—None	2—Moans to pain	3—Flexion to pain
	1—None	2—Extension to pain
		1—None

Bilirubin Nomogram

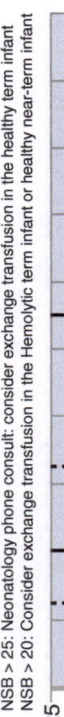

NSB > 25: Neonatology phone consult: consider exchange transfusion in the healthy term infant
NSB > 20: Consider exchange transfusion in the Hemolytic term infant or healthy near-term infant

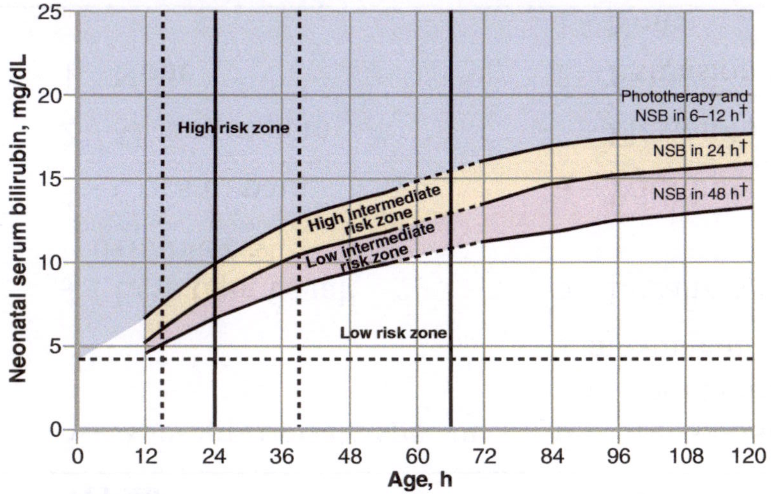

Risk factors
- Jaundice in the first 24 h
- Visible jaundice before discharge
- Previous jaundiced sibling
- Gestation ≤ 38 weeks
- Exclusive breastfeeding

- East Asian race
- Bruising cephalophematoma
- Maternal age > 25 years
- Male gender

†A TcB may be substituted for NSB. Near exchange levels, a NDB is preferred
NSB = Neonatal serum bilirubin; TcB = Transcutaneous bilirubin

Pediatric Head CT Criteria

Age <2 years (<3 months = CT)

	CT	Observe or CT
AMS or GCS <14	Yes	
Skull FX	Yes	
Scalp hematoma		Yes
LOC >5 s		Yes
Not normal per parent		Yes

Age >2 years

	CT	Observe or CT
AMS or GCS <14	Yes	
Skull FX	Yes	
h/o LOC		Yes
h/o Vomiting		Yes
Headache		Yes

Adapted from: Kuppermann N et al. Identification of children at very low risk of clinically-important brain injuries after head trauma: A prospective cohort study. *Lancet* 2009 Sep 15

Sick Neonate "THE MISFITS"

- Trauma
- Heart disease/congenital
- Endocrine/electrolyte
- Metabolic
- Inborn errors of metabolism
- Sepsis
- Formula (too dilute/concentrated)
- Intestinal catastrophe
- Toxins
- Seizures

Pediatric Fever Neonate

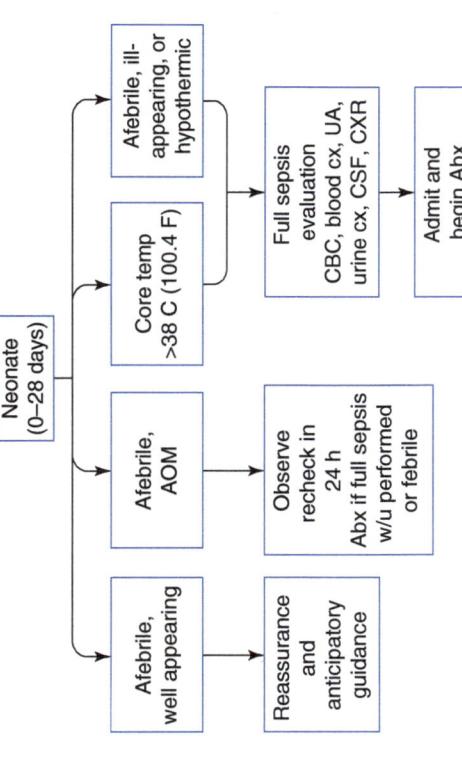

Adapted from Pediatric Emergency Medicine Reports, Hernandez and Nguyen "Fever in Infants <3 Months Old: What is the Current Standard?"

Pediatric Fever (1–2 Month Old Infant)

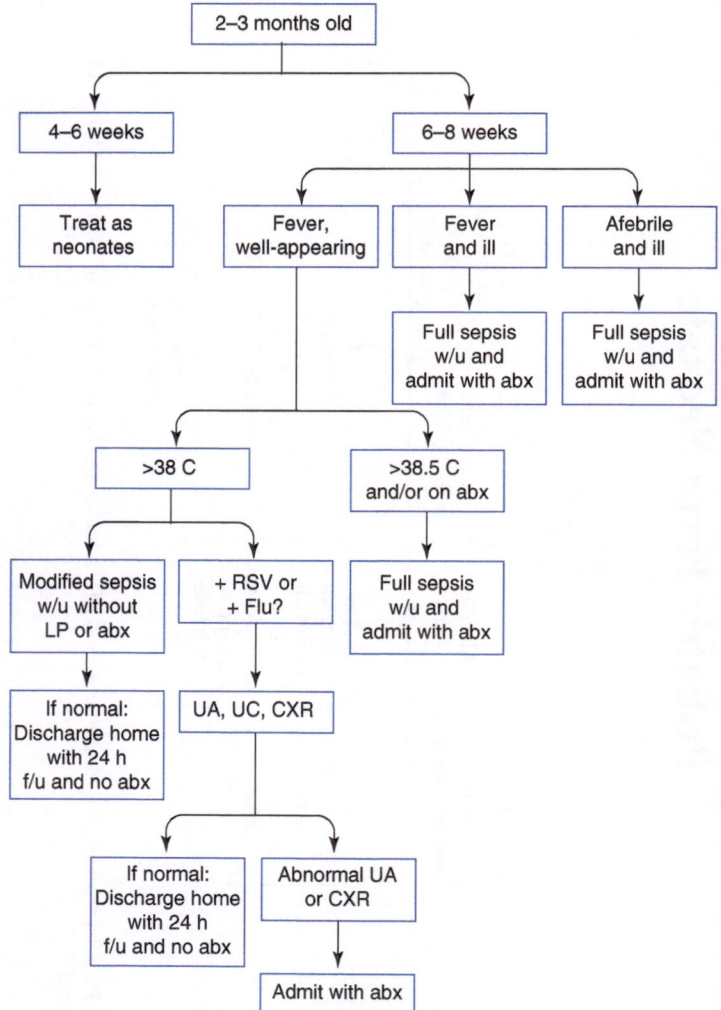

Adapted from Pediatric Emergency Medicine Reports, Hernandez and Nguyen "Fever in Infants <3 Months Old: What is the Current Standard?"

Pediatric Fever (2–3 Month Old Infant)

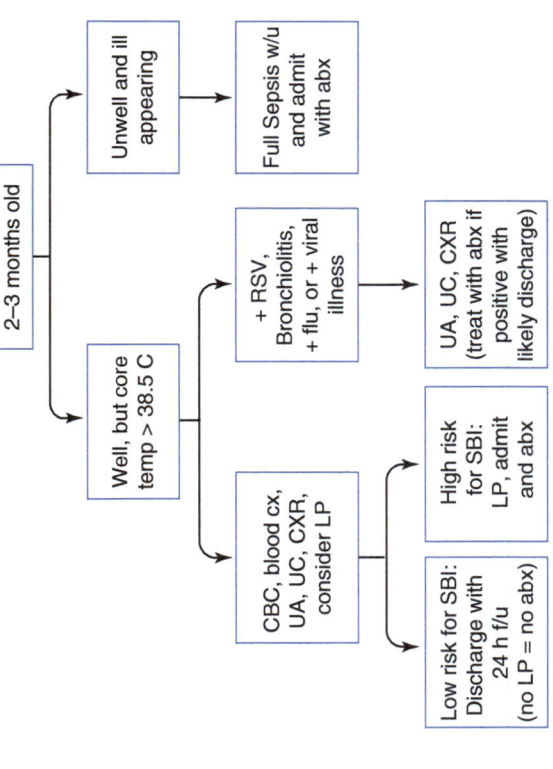

Adapted from Pediatric Emergency Medicine Reports, Hernandez and Nguyen "Fever in Infants <3 Months Old: What is the Current Standard?"

Pediatric Abdominal Pain

Neonate	2 months to 2 years	2–5 years	Over 5 years
Malrotation with midgut volvulus	Non-accidental trauma	Non-accidental trauma	Non-accidental trauma
Pyloric stenosis	Incarcerated hernia	Appendicitis	Appendicitis
Necrotizing enterocolitis	Intussusception	Intussusception	Diabetic ketoacidosis
Testicular torsion	Hirschsprung disease	Ovarian torsion	Sickle cell syndrome
			Vaso-occlusive crisis
	Meckel's diverticulum	Hemolytic uremic syndrome	Ovarian torsion
	Hepatitis	Meckel's diverticulum	Cholecystitis
			Pancreatitis
			Hemolytic uremic syndrome

19

Head and Neck

B. Allen et al., *Quick Hits in Emergency Medicine*,
DOI 10.1007/978-1-4614-7037-3_19,
© Springer Science+Business Media New York 2013

Modified Centor (McIsaac) Criteria for Evaluation of Pharyngitis

Points	Total score and risk
1	−1 or 0 (1 %)
1	1 (10 %)
1	2 (17 %)
1	3 (35 %)
1	4 (>50 %)
−1	5 (>50 %)

If score 1–3, get rapid test

If score >4, treat empirically

Adapted from McIsaac, WJ et al. Empirical Validation of Guidelines for the Management of Pharyngitis in Children and Adults. JAMA. 2004 April 7; 291:1587–1595

Retropharyngeal Abscess

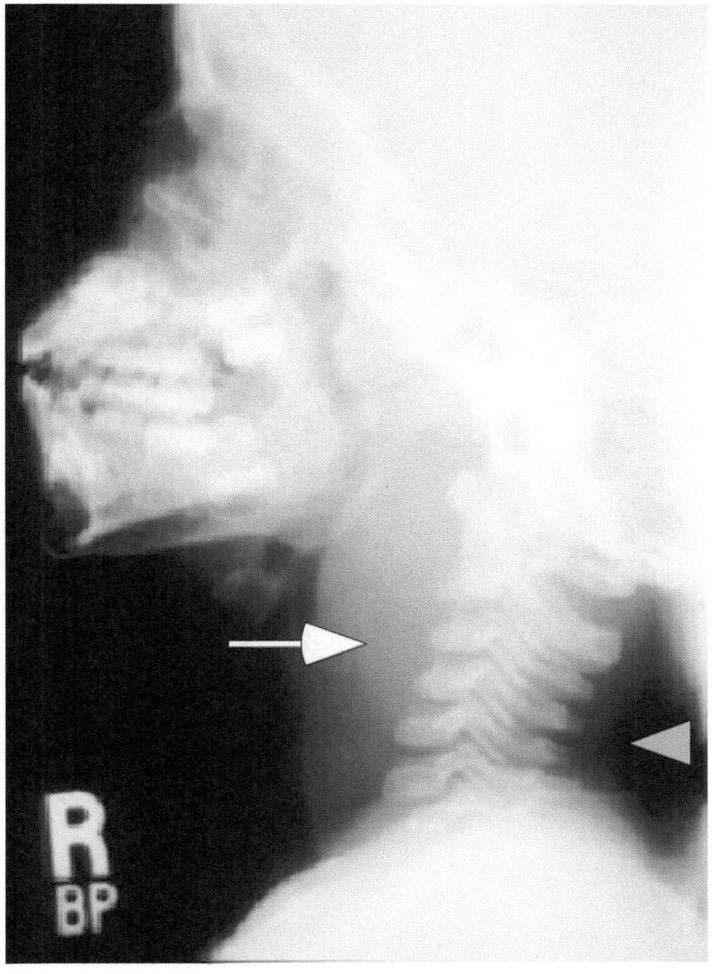

*Solid arrow represents large amount of prevertebral edema
*Dashed arrow represents air
Used with permission from first aid for the emergency medicine clerk-
ship, 3rd Ed., by Stead et al., McGraw Hill

Epiglottitis

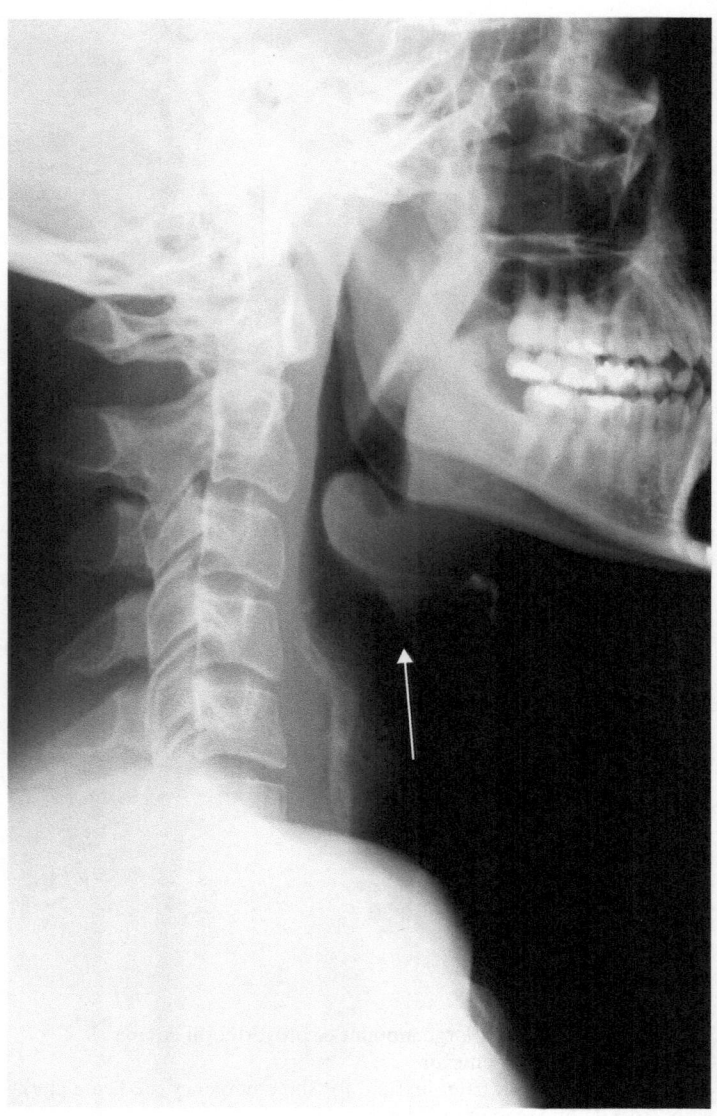

From first aid for the emergency medicine clerkship, 3rd Ed., by Stead et al., McGraw Hill

20

Statistics

B. Allen et al., *Quick Hits in Emergency Medicine*,
DOI 10.1007/978-1-4614-7037-3_20,
© Springer Science+Business Media New York 2013

Statistics

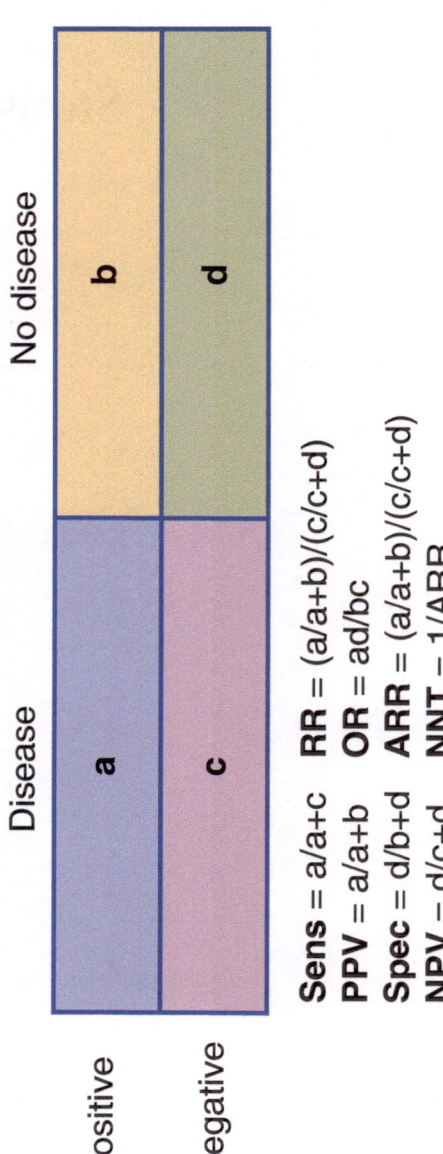

	Disease	No disease
Positive	a	b
Negative	c	d

Sens = a/a+c   **RR** = (a/a+b)/(c/c+d)
PPV = a/a+b   **OR** = ad/bc
Spec = d/b+d   **ARR** = (a/a+b)/(c/c+d)
NPV = d/c+d   **NNT** = 1/ARR

Sens sensitivity, *Spec* specificity, *RR* relative risk, *ARR* adjusted relative risk, *PPV* positive predictive value, *NPV* negative predictive value, *OR* odds ratio, *NNT* number needed to treat

21

Infusions, Pressors, and RSI

B. Allen et al., *Quick Hits in Emergency Medicine*,
DOI 10.1007/978-1-4614-7037-3_21,
© Springer Science+Business Media New York 2013

Medications and Infusions

		Push Dose Pressors
Amiodarone	1 mg/min × 6 h	Epinephrine (1:10,000 = 1 mg/10 ml)
	0.5 mg/min × 18h	1 cc epi and 9 cc NS=1:100,000=10 mcg/ml
Decadron	0.6 mg/kg (10 mg max)	Administer 0.5–2 cc IV q2–5 min
Dopamine	5–20 mcg/kg/min	
Dobutamine	5–20 mcg/kg/min	
Epinephrine	0.05–1 mcg/kg/min	
Epinephrine SC	0.1–0.5 mg SQ	
Esmolol	500 mcg/kg for 1 min	
	50–100 mcg/kg/min	
Fentanyl	1 mcg/kg/min	
Labetalol	0.5–2 mg/min	
Lasix	0.25–0.75 mg/kg/h	
Levophed	1 mcg/min	
Mannitol	1–2 g/kg	
Nitroglycerine	5–20 mcg/min	

Nitroprusside	0.5–4 mcg/kg/min	
Pentobarb	1 mg/kg/h (1–5 mg/kg load)	
Phenylephrine	0.1–10 mcg/kg/min	Phenylephrine (10 mg/ml)
Procainamide	3–6 mg/kg over 5 min	1 cc = 10 mg
	20–80 mcg/kg/min	Injection into 100 cc NS = 100mcg/ml
Propofol	10 mcg/kg/min titrate	Administer 0.5–2 cc IV q2–5 min
Vasopressin	0.01–0.04 units/min	
Versed	0.02–0.1 mg/kg/h	
RSI		
Etomidate	0.3 mg/kg	
Ketamine	2 mg/kg	
Lidocaine	1–1.5 mg/kg	
Rocuronium	0.5–1 mg/kg	
Succinylcholine	1–1.5 mg/kg	
Vecuronium	0.1 mg/kg (0.01 defasc)	
Versed	0.1 mg/kg	

Errata

Quick Hits in Emergency Medicine

Brandon Allen, Latha Ganti and Bobby Desai

B. Allen et al., *Quick Hits in Emergency Medicine*,
DOI 10.1007/978-1-4614-7037-3,
© Springer Science+Business Media New York 2013

DOI 10.1007/978-1-4614-7037-3_22

The publisher regrets that in the print and online versions of this book the following errors occurred. See the next page for the corrections.

The online version of the original chapter can be found at
http://dx.doi.org/10.1007/978-1-4614-7037-3

B. Allen et al., *Quick Hits in Emergency Medicine*,   E1
DOI 10.1007/978-1-4614-7037-3,
© Springer Science+Business Media New York 2013

1

ACLS

Page 3

In the lower right-hand box, "Epineprine" should be spelled "Epinephrine"

The online version of the original chapter can be found at
http://dx.doi.org/10.1007/978-1-4614-7037-3_1

3

Sepsis and Resuscitation

Page 15

In the table under Early Goal-Directed Therapy, "prossors" should be spelled "pressors"

The online version of the original chapter can be found at
http://dx.doi.org/10.1007/978-1-4614-7037-3_3

19

Head and Neck

Page 120

The correct table for Modified Center (McIsaac) Criteria is the following:

MODIFIED CENTOR (McISAAC) CRITERIA

Clinical feature	Points	Total score and risk
h/o fever or temp > 38 C	1	−1 or 0 (1 %)
Absence of cough	1	1 (10 %)
Tender anterior cervical nodes	1	2 (17 %)
Tonsillar swelling or exudates	1	3 (35 %)
Age < 15	1	4 (>50 %)
Age > 45	−1	5 (>50 %)
If score < 0 don't treat;	If score 1–3 get rapid test;	If score > 4 treat empirically

Adapted from McIsaac, WJ et al. Empirical Validation of Guidelines for the Management of Pharyngitis in Children and Adults. JAMA. 2004 April 7; 291: 1587–1595

The online version of the original chapter can be found at
http://dx.doi.org/10.1007/978-1-4614-7037-3_19

Index

B. Allen et al., *Quick Hits in Emergency Medicine*,   129
DOI 10.1007/978-1-4614-7037-3,
© Springer Science+Business Media New York 2013